It's All
Good Hair

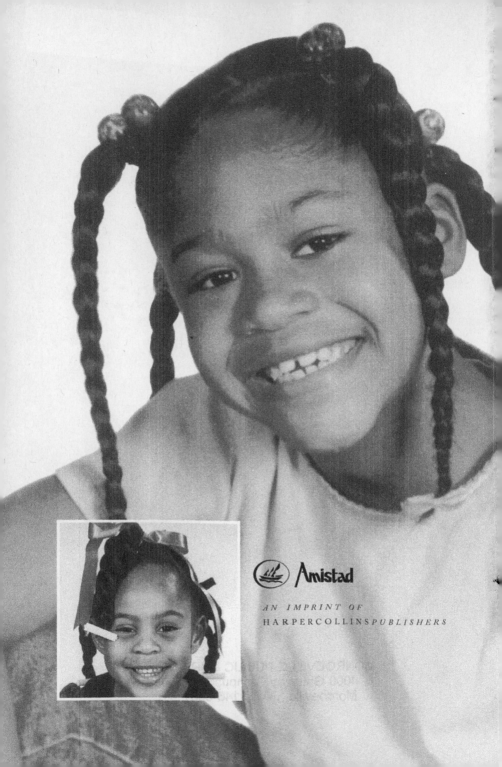

Amistad

AN IMPRINT OF
HARPERCOLLINSPUBLISHERS

It's All Good Hair

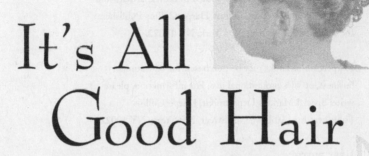

THE GUIDE TO STYLING AND GROOMING BLACK CHILDREN'S HAIR

Michele N-K Collison

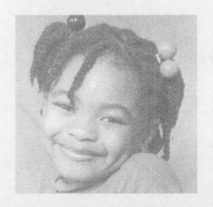

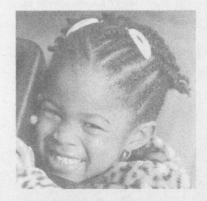

HarperCollins books may be purchased for educational, business, or sales promotional use. For information, please write: Special Markets Department, HarperCollins Publishers Inc., 10 East 53rd Street, New York, NY 10022.

FIRST EDITION

DESIGNED BY DEBORAH KERNER /
DANCING BEARS DESIGN

Printed on acid-free paper

Library of Congress Cataloging-in-Publication Data
Collison, Michele N-K
It's all good hair: the guide to styling and grooming black children's hair/
Michele N-K Collison—1st ed.
p. cm.
ISBN 0-06-093487-5
1. Hairdressing of Blacks. 2. Hair—Care and hygiene.
3. Hairstyles. I. Title.
TT972. C59 2002
646.7'24—dc21   2001053573

14 15 ❖/RRD 20 19 18 17 16 15

TO MAYA
AND MICHAEL WILLIAMS—

MY BEAUTIFUL TWINS WHO
BROUGHT THIS BOOK TO LIFE

Contents

Acknowledgments

This book would not have been possible without the extraordinary support and time of a number of people. First I would like to thank my mother, Julie Collison-Careathers, for always telling me to dream big dreams and for always being there for me. My love and gratitude to my husband, Michael Williams, for his inspiration and support. To my dad, Sinclair Careathers, and my brother Michael, thanks for all your words of wisdom.

Much love to my fabulous friend, TaRessa Stovall, who first suggested that I stop talking about the fact that there was no book on African-American children's hair care and actually write one. To the divas, Cheryl and Niki, who were never more than a phone call away. My incredible agent, Djana Pearson Morris, who believed in me and got me my book deal. And my amazing editors, Manie Barron and Sarah Wharton, who saw the possibilities. To Rick, thanks for listening and for planting the seeds for a richer life.

Thank you to the incredibly talented Kea Prather, whose long hours and beautiful pictures made this book what it is. I cannot thank Jill Carpenter and Susan Peterkin-Bishop enough for creating such beautiful hairstyles on the girls and boys. My thanks to my longtime stylist, Tim Gray, and Billye Smith, for plain talk about hair, and to Marcy Walker, for explaining the difference between a flat twist and a two-strand twist. Kudos to Wesley Clark, who translated the hairstyles into wonderful illustrations. And I can't forget Dr. Valerie Callender, for her explanation of hair diseases.

Much gratitude to the moms and dads who gave so generously of their time and their children during the photo shoots. And to the models who looked so beautiful wearing their 'dos. Finally, love and kisses to my beautiful children, Maya and Michael Williams, whose hair inspired me to write this book in the first place.

Credits

Hair Models

JeNayc Alston

Alonzo Bailey

Sarah Bailey

Ngozi Bailey

Jordan Barksdale

Kamaria Beamon

Iyanu Bishop

Akayla Bracey

Carlton Bridgeforth

Randall Bridgeforth

Robyn Brittain

Camille Brittain

Morgan Dailey

Sydney Dailey

Sydney Friend

Alyssa Gill

Dara Gill

Rayvon Hebron

Aleah Jones

Justin Lane

Clay LaVeist

Kordaye McAllister

Carelle Macon

Joel Maxwell

Kerelle Maxwell

Nicole Mitchell

Sydney Mitchell

Johnny Parks

Sydney Pearson

Heather Phillips

Alexis Rickford

Kara Rickford

Delamica Robinson

Denzel Ruff

Joye Ruffin

Olivia Shields Dabre
Bambara

Mariah Stovall

Aja Taylor

Nickayla Tucker

Camille Wilson

Maya Williams

Photography

All photographs are by Kea Prather of Imagine Studios of Washington, D.C., except those of medical conditions, which are provided by Dr. Valerie Callender.

Illustrations

All illustrations are by Wesley Clark.

Hairstylists and Consultants

Hairstyles are by Jill Carpenter of Big G's Images, and Susan Peterkin-Bishop, Angela Maxwell, and Penny Jones of Jaah Studios (both studios located in Silver Spring, Maryland). Barber styles are by Shawn Hill of Shades Design of Silver Spring, and Delton Graham of Big G's Images (Silver Spring, Maryland), except the hairstyle of Joye Ruffin, which was done by Cornrows and Co., of Washington, D.C.

Additional hair consultation was by Tim Gray of Connie's Headquarters of Silver Spring, Maryland; and by Marcy Walker of Madame Walker's Braidery of Temple Hills, Maryland.

Introduction

What are you going to do with that child's hair? My friends started bombarding me with questions when my daughter Maya was around six months old. What did my friends mean when they asked what was I going to do with Maya's hair? I wasn't planning to do anything with her hair. I was a new mother of twins. Do hair? I just wanted to sleep. She was a baby and I let her hair be free. Her brother Michael's hair was even less of an issue. I'd use a soft brush on it occasionally.

But by the time Maya was a year old, it was clear that her free-spirited, curly Afro was not working anymore. I would have to do something with her hair. I decided to fall back on the tried-and-true: two neat braids with a part down the middle. The first time I tried to do her hair, I sat her on my lap, just as my mother had done with me. I had all the necessary equipment—the comb, the brush, the barrettes, and the pink oil.

I thought to myself, "I am a college graduate with all kinds of skills and talents. What's so hard about a part and a few braids?" Maya wasn't so sure. She was squirming during my frustrating attempts to get her hair in this simplest of styles.

Finally I was finished. All right, so her part was crooked and her braids were kind of lumpy. At least I had gotten it in a style. I was feeling pretty good about my efforts.

All that changed, though, when my mother came over, rolled her eyes, took one look at her granddaughter's head, and said, "Bring me that child." Fifteen minutes later, my mother had Maya looking like a child in a toothpaste commercial. Her hair was perfect, the braids were flawless, and not one strand of hair was out of place.

Watching my mother do Maya's hair, it seemed so simple and natural. Why then, was it so hard when I tried? My mother had learned from her mother, who learned from her mother. Braiding had been passed down from the people of Africa through their descendants in America. This tradition seemed to have skipped me. I don't even remember braiding my doll-baby's hair. And I couldn't remember the last time I had done my own hair. Ever since I got a job making decent money, I've had a standing weekly appointment with my hairdresser, Tim Gray.

My struggles to learn to do Maya's hair became a running joke. When my friends saw Maya, they laughed and said, "Michele must have done that child's hair." When I picked Maya up from daycare, she would have a new hairstyle every day. Her teacher would just do it over. Finally, she just said, "Bring me a brush and comb so I can do Maya's hair here."

When I would share my hair-care dilemmas with others, they would tell me to just cornrow her hair—as if all Black women are born knowing how to braid. But I was going to have to learn some braiding styles pretty quickly, or other mothers would be clucking their teeth over my poor daughter's hair. Black folks put a premium on nice-looking hair. You simply can't have your child walking around in the Black community with some raggedy-looking 'do.

Eventually, with the help of my mother, I learned how to do some decent ponytails. That worked for about two years. But by the time I mastered simple plaits, Maya raised the ante. My fashion-conscious daughter started demanding more elaborate hairstyles. "Mommy, I'm tired of wearing my hair in two ponytails," Maya would say. "I want my hair to look like that," she'd say as she pointed at the picture of a girl with some fancy braids swept up on her head. (It's amazing the faith children have in their mothers.) Maya didn't know that it was a major accomplishment that her mother had mastered braids. Nor did she know that I couldn't tell a flat twist from a cornrow.

Eventually I learned that I wasn't alone with my hair-care

drama. Many other Black mothers and fathers, and White and Biracial mothers, were also secretly ashamed that they don't know how to do their children's hair—folks who had law degrees but couldn't figure out how to make a straight part in their childrens' hair.

Conversation after conversation with Black parents and White parents with Biracial and Black children always turned to, "What do you do with your child's hair?" There are the tears and the drama associated with combing our children's gloriously curly locks. Half the battle in the mornings was trying to get the kids to sit still to get their hair done. My cousin Gina said it was always a struggle to do her daughter Tiara's hair. "First I have to find Tiara. Whenever she sees me pick up that comb, she runs away."

For some parents, the hair salon is their salvation. Mothers told me the way they avoided the hair drama was to schedule a weekly appointment for their young daughters at the salon, some as young as two and three years old. Even though their daughters' hair was done, these mothers still said they felt they should know how to style their own children's hair.

The Broken Link?

For a variety of reasons, many of today's African-American parents have no idea how to properly care for their children's hair. For centuries, Africans have been recognized for their intricate braiding styles. And African-American women have vivid memories of sitting between their mothers' or grandmothers' knees as they put Dixie Peach or Blue Beaugamont in our hair. We laugh as we remember sitting in the kitchen listening to the hiss of the straightening comb and twisting in our seats when the relaxer started to burn.

But those basic hairdressing skills got lost somewhere along the way. Mostly, these skills didn't seem very important next to listening to Earth, Wind and Fire or running track in junior high and high school. My friends and I didn't sit around doing each other's hair, and we didn't spend any time playing with dolls. As soon as we got old enough, we'd rush to the hairdresser to get our hair done. We barely knew how to do our own hair.

By the time we started having our own kids there was no one around to help us untangle this hair stuff. Today Grandma and Aunt Betty are half a continent away or too busy working to teach Hair Care 101. So we depend on the teenage girl down the street to come twice a week to fix up Ashely's hair. And we admire the styles on other girls. But who can tell a flat twist from a double-strand twist? And who has time to learn? And even if you had time, where would you go to learn?

And it's not just Black women who are looking for some basic hair-care instructions. More single fathers are raising their daughters and desperately trying to figure out the hair thing. And as old taboos over race continue to fall, people are marrying partners of different ethnicities and having children with radically different hair textures than their own. If your hair texture is straight and blond what are you going to know about taking care of a little girl with short, kinky hair? One White mother was so desperate for some basic information she followed my girlfriend around a CVS drugstore asking questions about what shampoo and hair oil to use on her adopted African-American daughter's head.

Today, Black people feel they have freedom to style their hair any way they wish. We now see locks, braids, twists, Afros, relaxed styles, curly 'dos. Even though we are seeing more styling choices, the "good-hair-bad-hair" thing is still with us. Remember the outcry a few years ago over the White teacher in New York who thought she was teaching her mostly Black schoolchildren to appreciate their hair when she assigned the book *Nappy Hair*. Black people had been dealing with these demons for years, but suddenly the rest of the country had "stumbled on our race secret," said journalist Jill Nelson. "Black folks hated their hair."

Black children are introduced to this color caste system early, leaving psychological scars that last for life. Many young Black girls grow up feeling as Maya Angelou did when she wrote in her autobiography, *I Know Why the Caged Bird Sings*: "I was going to look like one of the sweet little white girls who were everybody's dream of what was right with the world. . . . Wouldn't they be surprised when one day I woke out of my black ugly dream, and my real hair, which was long and blond, would take the place of the'kinky mass that Momma wouldn't let me straighten."

Thankfully, my brother and I managed to escape much of this madness until we came to live in America. We were born overseas and had spent our early years in Ghana, where my father is from. Later on, my mother tells me a funny story about my hair when I was a baby. While she was in Germany, she and another friend of hers were pregnant around the same time. Her friend's daughter was born a few months earlier than I was. The baby was born with almost no hair and as it grew in, my mother said her friend constantly complained about how "bad" the child's hair was. When I was born a few months later with a head full of hair, my mother said her friend used to tell her that after my hair "turned," my hair would be nappy, too. Every night after that, my mother said she would pray over my head while she brushed it.

Maybe it was the crowd of locked, braided, and natural-wearing women I hung out with, but I naively thought the "good-hair-bad-hair" thing was over—until I had my children. As soon as my twins were born, the speculation started about what grade of hair those babies would have. Perfect strangers told me that I might be lucky, Maya's and Michael's hair might not turn. They might, in fact, keep that "good grade of hair."

I tried to shush these people. I told them this was a new day. We didn't talk about "good and bad hair." They didn't pay me any mind and kept on talking. Good hair, bad hair—I was just happy they had hair. But obviously this obsession was here to stay.

It didn't end there. One day Maya and Michael were on the playground when a little girl walked up to them and started admiring their hair. She said, "Ooh your children have such pretty hair." I smiled and told her that her hair, which was in two braids, was also pretty. "No it's not," she replied. "I have bad hair. Not like their hair. They have sexy hair, like on the videos." Although I repeatedly tried to point out to her that everybody had good hair, she was adamant. Short of a miracle, this child would grow up to believe that she was less attractive because she did not have long, flowing hair like the women who dance in music videos.

Our children come in a rainbow of hues and with all different types of hair—curly, kinky, wavy, straight, short, long, relaxed, locked. But all of our children's hair is beautiful, and we must begin to tell our children so. And we can begin by finding hairstyles that look good on our children's hair. There was nothing so inspiring as to see twenty little girls beaming into mirrors and exclaiming, "My hair is so beautiful" at the photo shoots for this book. The hairstyles weren't terribly complicated, and we worked to find hairstyles that flattered each child's face and hair texture. In reading the pages of this book, I hope that you will find a lot of information that helps you end the daily hair-care drama and make peace with your children's hair.

When I went looking for a book on Black children's hair six years ago, I couldn't find one. I looked in those Black beauty magazines you see at every grocery store. Usually they just had a bunch of photos of the latest celebrity hairstyles. Sometimes I'd get excited because there would be a few pictures of little girls with cute hairstyles. But the photos never had any directions! Now I know I can't just look at a photo of a hairstyle and turn around and make it work on Maya's hair. And I don't think most parents can, either. So I enlisted the help of a couple of hairstylists and barbers who patiently showed me several basic hairstyles.

This book will teach you the secret to a neat part and how to comb your child's hair without all the tears and drama. And while we all wore our hair in two pigtails when we were girls, those styles are old school now. Today our kids want twists, locks, and Afros. Thanks to the step-by-step instructions, you can learn how to do cornrows and double-strand twists. And for you moms who want to relax your daughter's hair, I'm not mad at you. I believe parents should have all kinds of hair-care options, and I've included tips and instructions to help you relax your child's hair safely.

I've talked to enough parents of Biracial children and parents who have adopted Black children to know the hair issue is driving many people crazy. Black children's hair texture is so different from that of White children's that so many people are tempted to just cut if off, or snatch it back into a ponytail. Don't give up. I'll explain hair textures and different hair products to make your life easier. The book also explains why Black hair needs oil, and offers hairstyles that will help cut down your stress level from the hair drama.

Dads who may be caring for their children for the first time might be overwhelmed by their daughter's hair. I'll give you tips on simple hairstyles that will get you out the door faster and helpful hints on good grooming habits. Fathers who do their daughter's hair say that their braiding sessions have brought an unexpected dividend—a way for them to bond with their girls.

And those of you who have boys know that you have hair issues, too. Like the never-ending search for the perfect barber who will cut your son's hair the way you want it cut. Perhaps your son's Afro is looking a little raggedy, and you want to know what to do to make it neater.

You don't need to be an expert to learn how to do the styles in this book. We only included styles that could be done by the average mother or father. Some of the hairstyles are really easy. Others take a little practice. I bought one of these mannequins at a beauty supply store and sat down to learn how to do cornrows. You'll be rewarded by the smiles on your children's faces when they realize that doing hair becomes less of a hassle and that they end up with a great new look.

But more important than the hip new hairstyles, I hope you take away the message that it is important to turn your combing and brushing sessions into loving experiences. While you comb and brush your child's hair, tell her how beautiful she looks. Also tell her how much you like combing her hair. Too often Black girls have to hear how "bad" their hair is or how unattractive they are.

My girlfriend Joye has a wonderful ritual that she started with her daughter Jordan when she turned two. After washing her hair, she and Jordan stand in front of a mirror and chant: "I am BEAUTIFUL! I am SMART!" More than anything, Joye wants Jordan to know that her beauty does not come from her hair.

I used to be depressed over all this obsession with good hair and bad hair, until my friend Jackie told me how she put a stop to this obsession over hair. Her husband came from a family that placed a premium on good hair. In fact, this was how they described people, Jackie said. "They would say, 'You know so-and-so, the one with the good hair.'" Before they had children, Jackie told her husband that there is no such thing as "good hair" and "bad hair." "It's all good hair," Jackie says she told him. "If there's hair growing on top of a person's head, that is good hair. Now if there's no hair growing, that's bad hair and we have a problem. Otherwise, all hair is good hair."

1 Pregnancy and Infant Hair Care

MAKING THE GRADE

When my daughter Sydney was born, everybody wanted to know who she looked like. They weren't asking about her eyes. They wanted to know what Black folks always want to know when a baby who can go either way on these things is born. Whose color is she? What kind of hair does she have?

The hair can be a tricky thing. Nothing for that but to wait a few months until the grade comes in good.

My paternal grandmother is a very light-skinned woman with straight hair and Black features. She had an inspection ritual she performed on all new babies in the family. A careful once-over to check for color and clarity before she pronounced judgment. I didn't know this until I introduced her to Sydney when she was about six months old.

She sat my baby on her lap. After a few minutes, she announced her findings. "Well her color is good. And her hair ain't half bad considering how Black that [Negro] is you married."

—LONNAE O'NEAL PARKER,
EXCERPT FROM AUGUST 8, 1999,
WASHINGTON POST ARTICLE

Pregnancy and Relaxers

There you are, reveling in your pregnancy, looking at the sonogram, and trying to get over morning sickness. Your skin is glowing and your hair has never looked better. Then at one of your prenatal visits, your doctor utters some astonishing words. "No relaxers while you are pregnant." "Wait a minute," you say, "not only do I have to look like a whale for nine months. I can't even wear my usual fly do while I'm pregnant?"

Stylists report that they see many women get their hair braided because their doctors have told them to stop relaxing their hair while they are pregnant. Women may get different advice from their doctors about whether to get a relaxer put in their hair while they are pregnant. Some doctors worry about whether relaxers may harm unborn children. Other doctors don't see any reason for concern and tell their patients to keep getting their touch-ups during their pregnancy. A study of 526 pregnant women by the Centers for Disease Control in 1999 found that women who used relaxers in their hair didn't stand a greater chance of delivering premature babies or smaller babies than women who didn't have relaxers in their hair.

However, the researchers urged that more research be done on pregnant women and relaxers. If you have any concerns, see your doctor.

Infant Hair Care

It's tempting to believe that Black people have come to love their curly locks. After all, we see celebrities like singer Lauryn Hill proudly wearing locks and basketball superstars like Alan Iverson still sporting braids.

But Black people are still obsessed with good and bad hair. If you don't believe it, eavesdrop on any conversation involving Black babies. The nappy patrol starts the inspections when the baby is born. Parents look at their babies and joke, "Ooh look at the beautiful curly hair. Too bad it's going to *turn* nappy in a couple of months." I've seen mothers wondering whether they could head off this disaster. I overheard one mother invoking her ancestors when she told another mother that her baby daughter would keep her good hair texture:

Mother One: "Girl, that hair is going to turn nappy."

Mother Two: "No it's not. It's going to stay straight like this because my grandmother was half Indian and she had hair like this."

Doctors and stylists agree that most Black children's hair texture will change over the first year of a baby's life. Their hair may grow out and be replaced by a different texture of hair. My son, Michael, was born with a full head of hair, then, at about six months, it grew out and was replaced by hair that just covered his scalp. Black babies are born bald, with little hair, or with a full head of hair. But the curly or straight hair that Black babies are born with is usually replaced by thicker, tightly curling locks, starting at six months of age.

And don't worry if your child's hair isn't growing as fast as you would like. Dr. Valerie Callender, a dermatologist who practices in Mitchellville, Maryland, says parents are concerned that their baby's hair won't grow, and come to her looking for vitamins or products to make it grow faster. Her suggestion: Don't worry. Callender says it can take up to three years for babies to grow a full head of hair. And your child's hair texture and length may continue to change until he or she reaches eight years old.

During the first months, you don't have to do much more than run a wet washcloth over your baby's hair. Use a soft baby brush if you wish. But be careful when you are touching your baby's head. Her head is still growing.

Shampooing an Infant

When your baby is older, you can begin to give gentle shampoos. Do this after you have bathed your child.

Use gentle baby shampoo. Look for one that is made for Black children's hair because other baby shampoos tend to dry the hair out.

1. Lay your baby in your arms and support his head. Using your hand or a small cup, wet the baby's head.

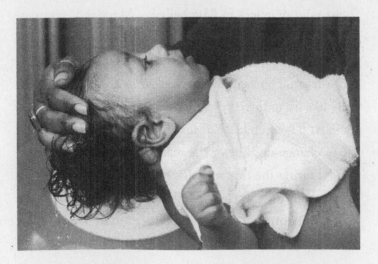

2. Rub a small amount of shampoo on his head. Using your fingertips, massage the shampoo on his scalp.

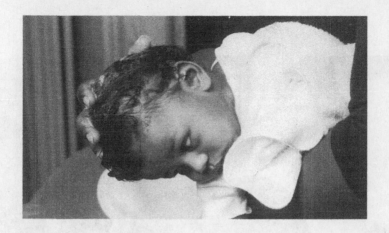

3. Rinse his head with the cup, being careful not to let any shampoo suds get into his eyes.

4. Use a soft towel to dry his hair.

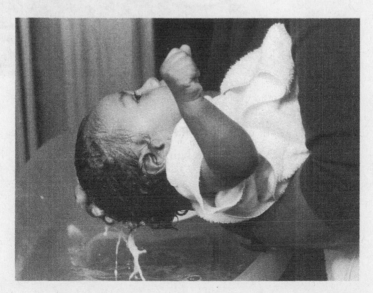

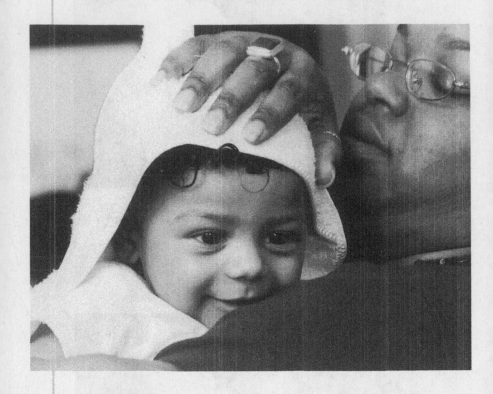

5. If you wish, use a light hair oil on his hair and a soft baby brush to style the hair.

Infant Hair-Care Tips

During the hot months, use a small baby hat to protect your baby's head from the hot sun. When it's cold outside, find a comfortable cotton or wool hat to keep your baby's head covered.

Stylist Susan Peterkin-Bishop suggests that you don't fuss too much with your baby's head. If you buy ornaments for your baby's hair, make sure they are not irritating your baby's head. "I see all these moms putting bows and ribbons in the baby's hair. Or the baby has patches of hair and they're trying to pull it all up into a ponytail. I just tell them to lighten up and enjoy their babies. They have plenty of time to do hair later on," she says. If you're at your wits' end and looking for something to do with your child's hair, turn to the later chapters for some styling suggestions.

Cradle Cap

One day, you may look at your baby and notice some white scaly patches on his scalp. This condition is called "cradle cap," and although it doesn't look attractive, it is not dangerous. Resist the temptation to pick at it or scrape it off, says Dr. Callender. Scraping it off will only irritate your child's scalp. Use some olive oil or baby oil to help loosen the flakes. Then shampoo your baby's hair with a gentle baby shampoo.

If the cradle cap gets thicker or moves down below your baby's ears or neck, consult your pediatrician or dermatologist.

2 Grooming

HAIR CUT

I adopted Jessica as a baby. Jessica is Biracial; her birth mother is White and her birth father is Black. When I was adopting Jessica, all the talk was about parenting issues, everything but her hair. I'm a White woman with straight hair, so I didn't know anything about how to do Jessica's hair. When Jessica was a toddler, I would twist it into two ponytails held with barrettes. I was worried she'd pull the barrettes out at day care and put them in her mouth. So, when she was one

I decided to cut her hair because it was a lot easier to take care of (and she looked really cute!). White parents often cut their kids' hair at that age, and it's kind of a rite of passage, from toddler to kid. I had no idea that hair was such a big deal for Black people. Jessica's godmother, who is Black, had a nightmare that I had cut her hair. When I asked her advice, she told me that Black folks have this thing about long hair and would never cut a little girl's hair. She said, "Black people just don't cut girls' hair. It's just not done." But when she saw Jessica, she too laughed about the nightmare, and Jessica gets lots of compliments, from both Black and White folks.

As Jessica got older, she still didn't like to sit still, and we were both frustrated with spending a lot of time on hair in the morning before work and school. Since that first haircut, Jessica herself has decided to have short hair (like her sister!). It give her a lot of freedom, especially for swimming in the summer. Jessica's hair has beautiful curls, and the short haircut really brings out the curls and her big brown eyes—but sometimes she worries that she looks like a boy. So, now that she's in grade school, we're going to give longer hair another try, to see if it's important enough to her to be more patient with caring for her hair.

—AMY GOLDSTEIN

I t's tempting to skip right over this chapter and get to the good stuff—the pictures of the hairstyles in this book. But if you really want to make your life easier, take a few minutes to read over some of the basic grooming tips the hairstylists offered in this chapter. After all, the foundation of a good hairstyle is healthy, well-groomed hair.

Textures of Black Hair

B lack children and Biracial children have a variety of hair textures—from bone-straight to wavy to tightly coiled and everything in between. A child's hair texture depends on his or her genetic makeup. That's why your daughter may not have the same hair texture as you do. Her hair texture could be more like yours or the same as your husband's great-grandmother.

For years, Black people have obsessed over whether their child's hair was "good" or "bad." I think it is important to know what type of hair your child has, not to label it "good" or "bad," but to save you a lot of time and headaches in the future. For instance, although Black folks have labeled kinky hair as "bad hair," kinky hair is the ideal hair for today's popular cornrows, twists, and locks.

Hair texture crosses racial boundaries. Black children can have straight hair and White children can have kinky hair. No one hair texture is good or bad; all children's hair can be styled attractively.

The hair follicle is what determines whether your child's hair is curly, kinky, wavy, or straight. If you could look at different strands under a microscope, you could see that straight hair comes from a round follicle,

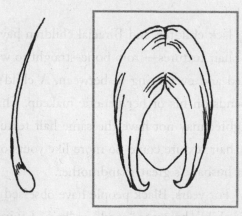

wavy hair from an oval follicle,

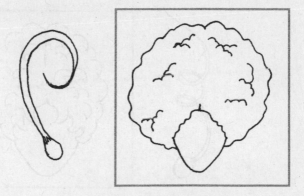

curly hair from a flat follicle,

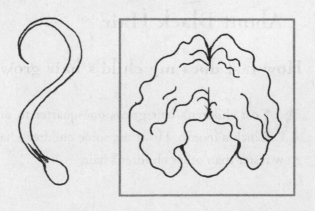

and kinky hair from a flat and spiraled follicle.

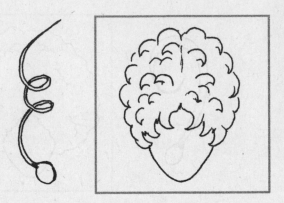

Common Questions About Black Hair

How fast does my child's hair grow?

Most children's hair grows one-quarter to one-half inch a month. However, some children's hair may grow faster than other children's hair.

Why won't my child's hair grow?

Your child's hair is growing, unless he or she has a medical problem (see chapter 10, "Hair Problems"). However, your child's hair may not be growing as long as he or she may like. Brushing, combing, and blow-drying all may take a toll on your child's hair and may be causing the hair to break before it can grow longer.

When you style your child's hair, consider parting the hair with your fingers or with a hair clip as shown in the picture below.

You may also consider twisting or locking your child's hair. Twists can be worn for two weeks at a time, while locking is permanent. When you twist and lock hair, you reduce the time needed to style it. When you

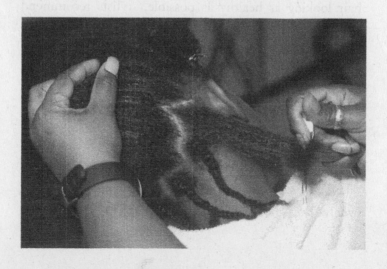

don't do anything to your child's hair, it can grow undisturbed.

Don't believe the hype about products that claim they will grow hair. You've seen the magazine ads featuring before-and-after pictures, the former showing short, damaged hair; the latter showing long, flowing hair. Doctors and stylists say that no product will make your child's hair grow. Invest your time and money instead in good habits and styling products.

Does my child need to get her hair trimmed?

I know that it is a capital crime to even suggest taking scissors to Black children's hair. But to keep your child's hair looking as healthy as possible, stylists recommend that you trim your child's hair every three months to get rid of split ends. If your child's ends look raggedy, and she frequently gets a lot of lint in her hair, she may need her hair trimmed. Split ends occur when the strand of hair starts to split because of combing, brushing, and blow-drying.

Don't try to trim your child's hair yourself. Instead, take her to a professional so that her hair will be trimmed evenly. But choose your stylist carefully, because some

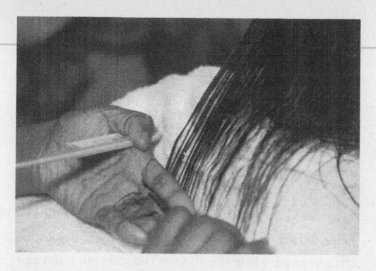

beauticians can get scissor-happy. A trim means cutting about one-sixteenth of the hair off the ends. A cut involves cutting a quarter inch or more of the hair.

What kind of brush and comb should I use?

The ideal tools to buy are a boar-bristle brush and a large-tooth comb.

How much moisture does Black hair need?

For years, Black folks have believed that all our hair problems can be solved with some hair grease or

Vaseline. If our child's hair was dry and brittle, we would just put some grease in it. Stylist Tim Gray says parents need to stop using petroleum jellies and baby oil to care for their children's scalp. Large amounts of these products just clog the scalp and do not allow the pores to breathe properly.

The scalp's natural sebaceous glands secrete oil that helps to keep the hair shaft lubricated. If your child has straight or wavy hair, the oil from the scalp can travel easily along the hair shaft. But oil needs a little help reaching the hair shaft of curly or kinky hair because it must negotiate the spiral coils to reach the end of the hair. So oiling your child's scalp every night is not going to do a whole lot for her hair.

Many hair manufacturers have recently made lighter hair oils for Black consumers. If your child's scalp is dry, you simply rub a small amount of hair oil in your hands and rub it over the hair.

How often do I need to shampoo my child's hair?

It depends on how dirty your child's hair becomes, but generally once a week or once every two weeks will suffice. Usually stylists don't recommend shampooing Black children's hair every day, because the shampoo will strip too much moisture from the hair.

Why are my baby's edges disappearing?

Stop braiding your child's hair so tight. You may also be guilty of putting relaxer on her "nappy edges" every three weeks to smooth them out. (If you want your child to have a hairline, read chapter 10, "Hair Problems.")

Are rubber bands bad for my child's hair?

Rubber bands can cause your child's hair to break. When you remove a rubber band from a child's hair, you will usually find a lot of hair stuck on the rubber band. To prevent hair breakage, use rubber bands that have a protective coating. When you remove the rubber bands, carefully cut them out of the child's hair with small scissors.

How does the weather affect my child's hair?

Parents know that weather can ruin a child's hairstyle. Rain can make your child's hair look frizzy. The humidity can make her hair puff out like a mushroom. Plan for the weather and try some of the hairstyles on the following pages that take advantage of the natural curl of your child's hair to minimize the effect of heat and moisture.

Shampoos and Conditioners

Admit it. You've been picking hair-care products based on what smells good or what was on sale at the drugstore. Stylists say a better bet would be to check out the pH balance on the back of the bottles. The pH balance tells the acidity or the alkalinity of a product.

Shampoos

L ook for a shampoo with a pH balance between 5 and 6.5. Many nationally advertised shampoo brands are designed to clean straight hair, which usually contains more oils than does kinky or curly hair. If you use shampoo that is too alkaline, you may shampoo away too much of the natural oil in your child's scalp and leave her hair feeling too dry. You may have to experiment with several products to find the ones that may work best for your child's hair type.

Check the pH balance on your baby shampoo also. It may cause your baby's hair to become too dry.

Some parents just grab the bar soap to shampoo their kids' hair. Stylists warn that bar soaps are not meant to be used as shampoo. They dry the hair out and leave a residue.

Conditioners

CREME RINSE

These are great to use right after you shampoo your child's hair to untangle it. The conditioner will also make her hair

23

softer by coating the cuticle, and it will add shine. Put it on your child's hair for a few minutes and then rinse it out.

MOISTURIZING CONDITIONER

These conditioners put moisture back into the hair by attracting and sealing water to the hair shaft. The conditioners also add moisture to your child's hair and add luster, making it easier to comb and style. These conditioners are most effective if you put a plastic cap on your child's head and place her under a hair dryer for 10 to 15 minutes. A heat cap can also be used.

RECONSTRUCTING CONDITIONER

These conditioners use proteins and nucleic acids to help strengthen dry, damaged hair. If your child's hair is really damaged, however, the best treatment may be the scissors.

HOT OIL TREATMENT

This treatment will add back to the hair some of the fatty acids that were removed during a chemical treatment or a process. However, hot oil treatments are not conditioners.

3 Braiding

ALL DAY WASH

It takes all day to wash my daughter JeNaye's hair. Her hair is so thick and long that it takes me, her daddy, and her big brother to get her hair done. Before we even get to the shampoo bowl, we have to bribe her with toys or candy. The candy usually works.

We have to lay her on her back on the counter. My husband supports her neck while singing silly songs or playing peek-a-boo or silly rhyming games—anything to distract her. I wash her hair, trying not to get any water in her ears. Water in the ears is a disaster because that means she'll want to get up and run. By the time I get to the second wash, JeNaye is repeating, "Are you finished, Mommy?" about five hundred times.

Here's where the fun really begins: now we have to comb her hair. The style she gets depends on her mood. If she is relaxed, we can be creative; if she's antsy, we do whatever is the fastest.

JeNaye hates to get her hair combed. She will try anything to stop the combing. Usually she says she needs to go to the bathroom or that her stomach hurts. These are stalling tactics. While I'm trying to do her hair, I let her watch, play, or eat anything she wants. I try to be careful not to pull her hair, but every tug of the comb is accompanied by a loud shriek. She will then flail her arms and throw the comb across the room and proceed to beg me not to use *that* comb! On several occasions she has cried to the point of vomiting. To calm her we again adhere to the wishes of JeNaye—whatever they may be. I have done her hair while she sits, lays, or hugs her dad. We have given her feasts of candy and juice. But about three hours into the ordeal we are about halfway through. After combing through her hair and oiling her scalp, it's time to style.

After a "style-tolerance check," I will determine if I'll do two ponytails, braids, or a combo of both, but it will all depend on how much the Queen can take. By now I am getting tired and Dad is running out of tricks and patience. Her brother (who lacks any attention during this process) has long asked "Are you done yet?" By the time we are finished, a total of five hours have passed. And we are all tired.

—ANGELA ALSTON

How many of us remember those Saturday-night hair rituals in the kitchen? We'd sit between our mother's or grandmother's knees while they lovingly oiled our scalps and braided our hair. Depending on how many sisters we had, this routine might last four or five hours. *Get real!* With Ashley's soccer practice and Jamal's basketball games, who has all day to do anyone's hair anymore?

If you're like most working Black parents, your children's hair is putting a serious crimp in your morning routine. Between getting the kids fed, dressed, and out the door to school, you probably have ten minutes to get their hair done. But those ten minutes are usually accompanied by shrieking and shouts of "*Ow,* Momma, that hurts!"

Finally, after fifteen minutes of wrestling, you have your daughter's hair in some kind of style. But her part is kind of crooked, those braids are lumpy, and what's with those strands of hair escaping from those barrettes?

This hairstyle is definitely not going to win you any brownie points with Ms. Eva at the Bright Star Daycare Center. As a matter of fact, you can rest assured Ms. Eva will have done your child's hair over to perfection by the time you pick her up after work in the evening.

If you could just learn a few simple hairstyles, your mornings would be much more relaxed and you would stop feeling so ashamed when Ms. Eva tells you how easy it is to do your child's hair.

Read and practice the following instructions and you'll be able to cut down on the hair drama in your house.

TIP . . . .

Turn your combing and brushing sessions into loving experiences. While you comb and brush your child's hair, tell her how beautiful she looks. Also tell her how much you like combing her hair. Too often, Black girls have heard how "bad" or how unattractive their hair is.

Many braiders and hairstylists say, often-times, when parents bring their children to salons to get their hair styled, parents say, "You've got to do something with this hair. I have never seen hair this bad." Before these professionals begin to style the hair of Black children, they lift these children up and tell them how beautiful they are and how beautiful their hair is. Telling your child how much you enjoy combing her hair will go a long way to helping her grow to see herself as a beautiful, confident person.

Preparation:
Combing and Shampooing

ITEMS YOU'LL NEED

Shampoo

Conditioner

Wide-tooth comb

Shower nozzle or a small bowl

Brush

Spray bottle for water

Light hair oil

Combing

With a wide-tooth comb, comb out your child's hair before you shampoo. This removes dirt and tangles, and makes the hair easier to manage after the shampoo.

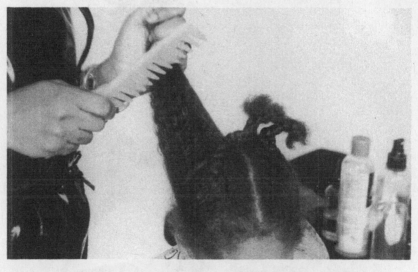

You can make combing hair less troublesome by combing from the ends first, then working your way to the roots. Hold your child's hair a half-inch from the end. Start combing through the ends of the hair. Not only is this quicker, because it removes the tangles first, it eliminates all the tugging and pulling that is caused by combing the hair from the scalp to the end of the strands.

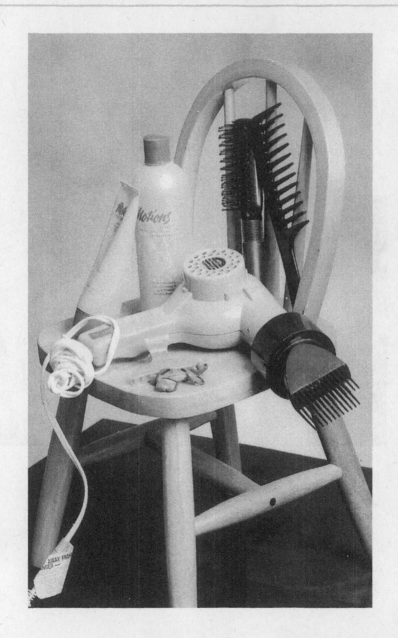

Shampooing Toddlers and Children

If your children are toddlers, you may want to wash their hair in the bathtub. Buy a shampoo cap to keep their faces from getting wet when you rinse their hair.

If your children are older, you will probably find it easier to shampoo their heads in the kitchen sink. Have your child lie face-up across the kitchen counter so you can wash her head in the kitchen sink. Place a towel underneath her neck.

If you don't have a counter, pull a chair up to the

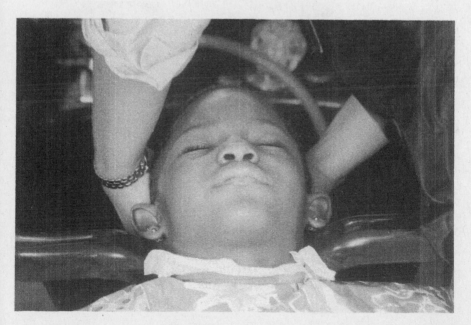

kitchen sink and let your child lean her head back into the sink. Place a towel under her neck to keep water from dripping down her back. (You may have to put a few telephone books or pillows under her so she can reach the sink.) You can also have her lean her head over the edge of the bathtub.

1. Before shampooing your child's hair, test the water to make sure it is not too hot. When the water is a comfortable temperature, rinse the hair well for two to three minutes.

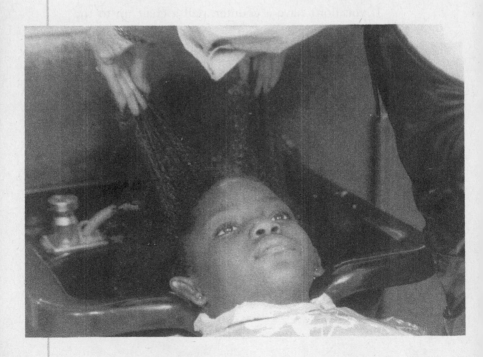

2. Place a bit of shampoo (about the size of a quarter) into your hand. Rub the shampoo between the palms of your hands. Starting from the nape of the neck and working your way to the ends of the hair, gently massage the shampoo in, using the balls of the fingers. Do not use your nails to scrub the scalp; scrubbing creates tangles and breaks the hair. During the shampoo, also massage the scalp thoroughly. Rinse the hair. There is no need to shampoo a second time; this strips hair of its natural essential oils and causes dryness and breakage.

3. After shampooing, use a moisturizing conditioner on the hair. It will also act as a detangler and will make the hair easier to comb. Put a bit of conditioner into your hand (again, about the size of a quarter), rub your palms together, and massage into the hair. Use a wide-tooth comb and comb the conditioner through the hair.

4. Put a plastic cap on your child's head and let her walk around or play for a bit (three to five minutes). This will allow the conditioner to penetrate the hair, making it softer and easier to comb. Rinse out the conditioner.

Shampooing is a very tiring experience for small children. Many stylists recommend that parents should wait a few minutes after shampooing, conditioning, and rinsing to style their children's hair, because small children will usually fall asleep. After your child goes to sleep, place the child on your lap, with her head facing you. While your little one sleeps, you can comb and brush the hair and put it in braids.

5. Try not to let your child's hair dry after shampooing because it will be harder to comb. Comb out the hair while it is wet. If some sections do become dry, use a water spray bottle to wet your child's hair. Use a wide-tooth comb to remove the tangles; fine-tooth combs will not allow you to comb through your child's hair well enough.

6. Part your child's hair into several sections and comb each section, working from the ends to the roots. When you have finished with each section of wet hair, twist it or braid it quickly before you go on to

the next section of hair. If you do this, your child's hair won't get tangled or matted while you comb the remaining sections of hair.

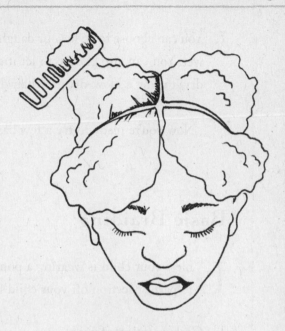

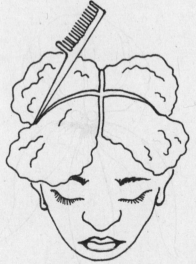

TIP . . . .

The secret to a neat part is a rat-tail comb. Take the long end of the comb and place the tip at the point on the scalp where you would like the part to begin. Gently draw it across the scalp and use the comb to separate the hair.

7. You can choose to style your daughter's hair while it is wet. You can also choose to let it air-dry naturally, or dry it using a blow-dryer or hair dryer.

Now you're ready to try a few basic styles:

Basic Braiding

Unless your child is wearing a ponytail, you will need to part or section off your child's hair.

1. Grab a section of hair and divide it into three even pieces. The secret to neat braids is to make sure you have three even pieces. If the sections of hair are uneven, the braids will be lumpy.

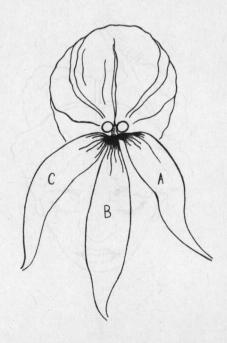

TIP . . . .

Most people braid over-handed; that is, you can see the backs of your hands while you braid. Over-handed braiding will create simple braids or what most of us call "plaits." However, the braids will not be as tight or last as long as those created by under-handed braiding.

2. Hold the three sections of hair in your hand. Place your thumbs on the right and left sections. Bring the right section under the middle, so the middle is now on the right. Your thumbs and your index finger should now make an X.

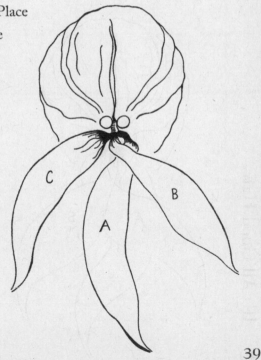

3. Now bring the left section under the middle section, so now the middle is on the left. Again, your thumbs and your index finger should make an X. Keep repeating this pattern until you have finished. You should now have a nice tight braid that should last for two or three days.

Once you have mastered this simple technique of under-handed braiding, you can move on to other hairstyles, since these braids serve as the foundation for several looks.

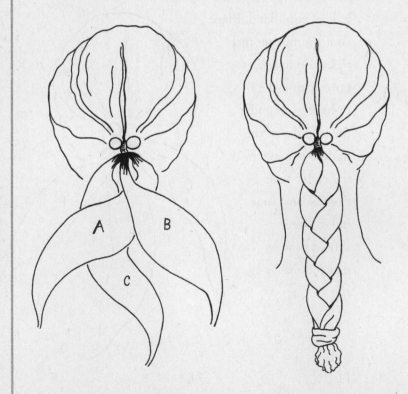

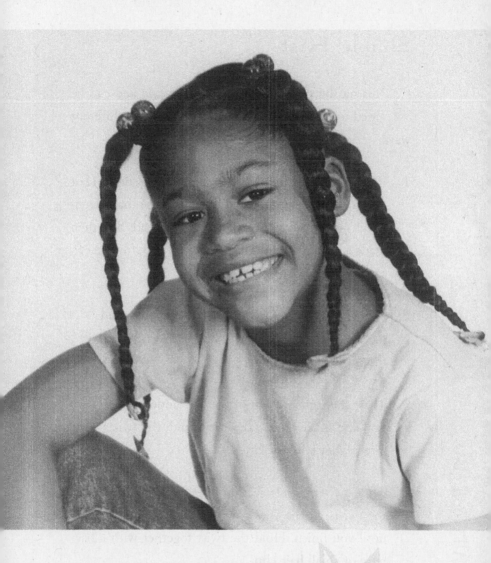

Simple Twists

This has become a very popular hairstyle and can be used to style your child's hair in a variety of different ways.

1. Part the hair in the desired number of sections. (For Aleah's hairstyle, stylist Jill parted the hair from Aleah's forehead to the center of her head. She then made a part in the middle of Aleah's head, from ear to ear.)

2. Gather a section of hair. Divide it into two even pieces. Hold the sections of hair between your thumbs and forefingers.

3. Twist the right section of the hair under the left section and make an X. (Be sure to pull the twists tight or else they will not last.)

4. Then twist the left section over the right. Continue the twists all the way down each section of the hair until you finish. Hold the twist together with a barrette or small hair clip.

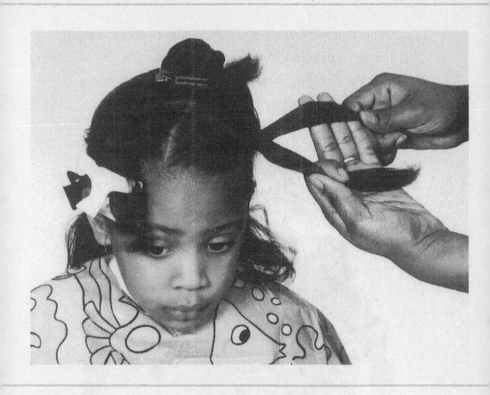

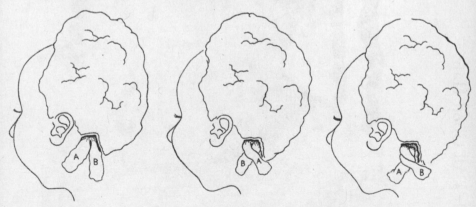

Now that you know how to do simple twists you can do unique variations. When your daughter needs to attend a dressier function, try any of these easy styles (instructions follow, beginning on page 47):

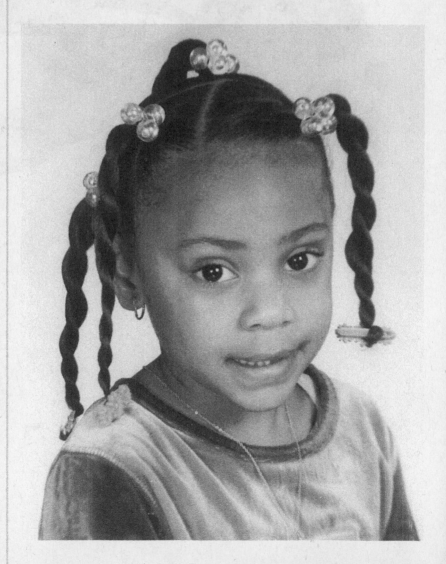

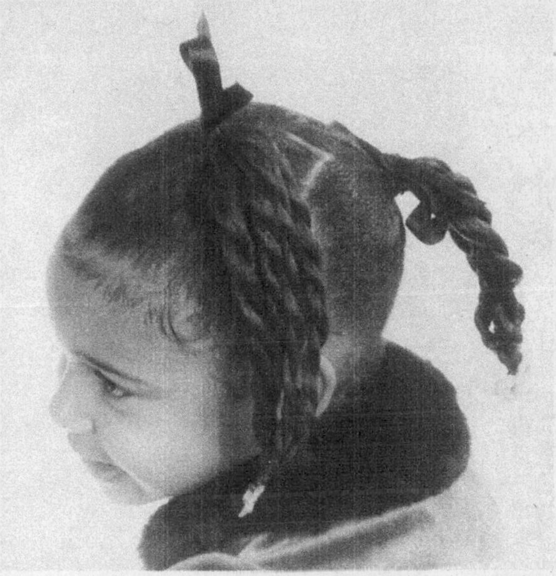

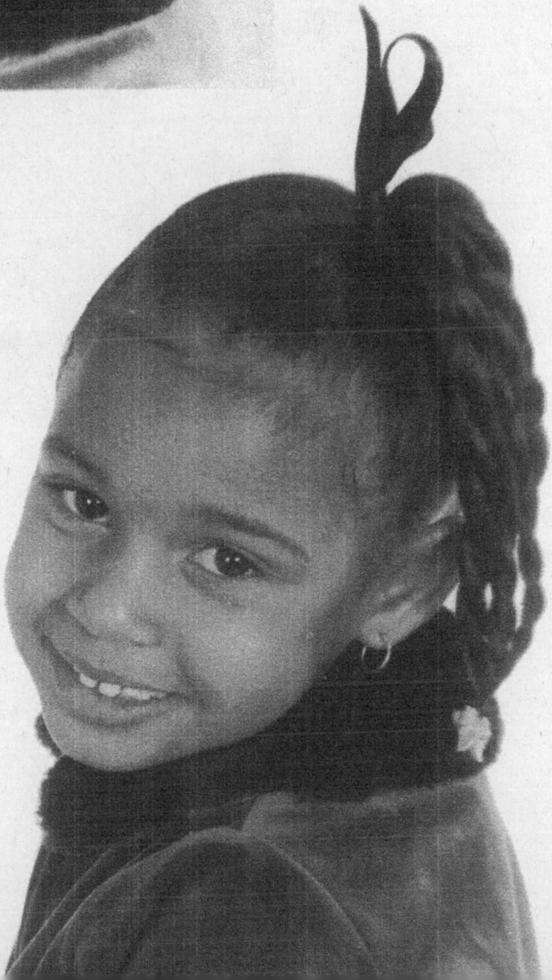

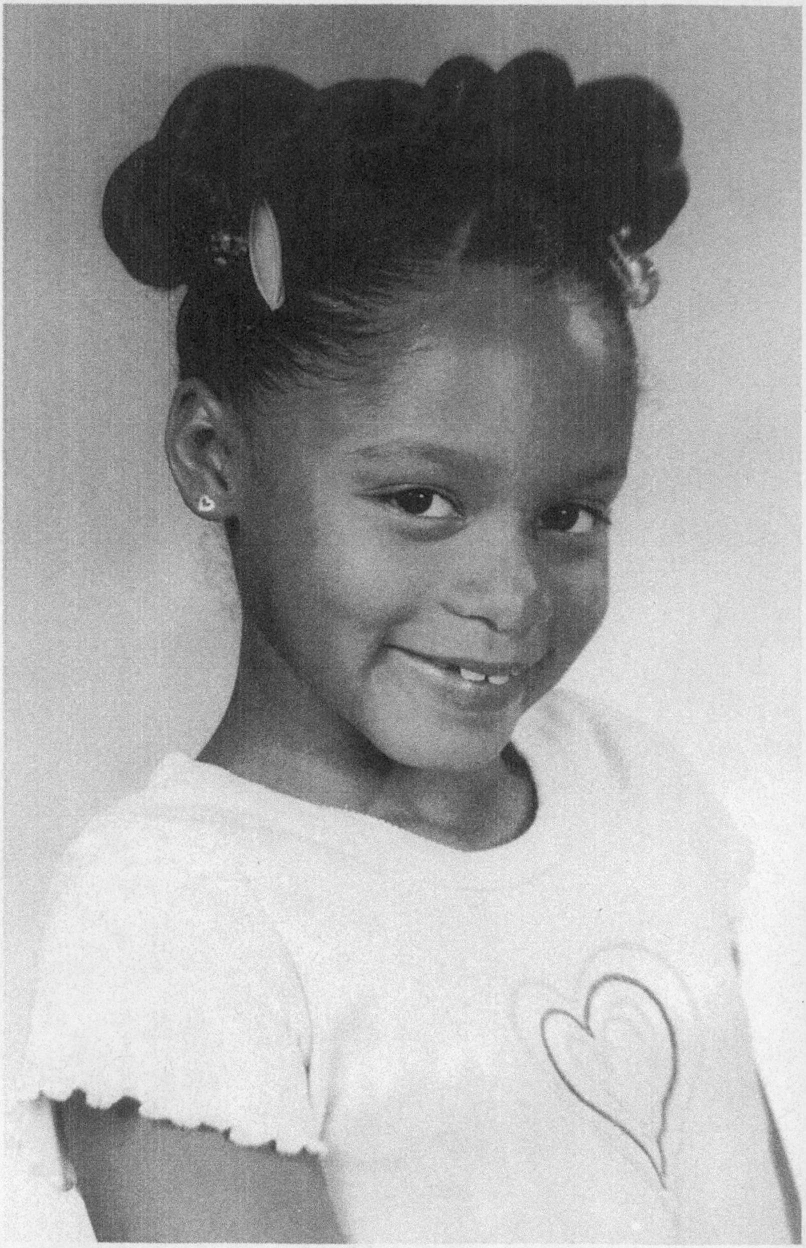

For hairstyle on page 45:

1. In one section of hair, make two or three ponytails, and then make two or three twists of each.

2. Then connect the ponytails at the ends with a plastic barrette.

3. Do this with a few sections of the head.

For hairstyle on page 46:

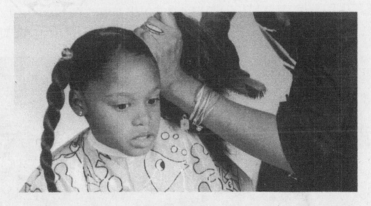

1. Brush the hair and section into two ponytails to the sides of the head.

2. Gather the hair from the head, and hold the hair together with a barrette or ponytail at the base of the head.

3. Make each ponytail into a twist; hold each twist at the end with a barrette or hair clip.

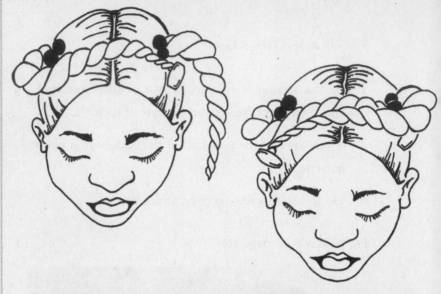

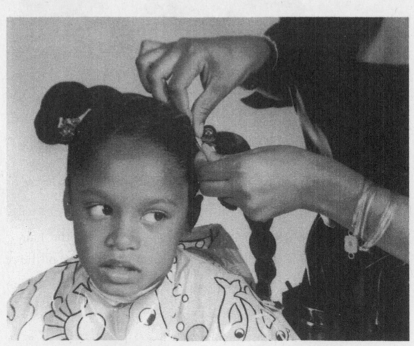

4. Fold one twist over to the other side of the head and, using the end barrette, attach the first twist to the head, clipping under the opposite twist.

5. Take the second twist and attach the end under the opposite twist, using the end barrette.

Instuctions for the hairstyle below begin on page 50.

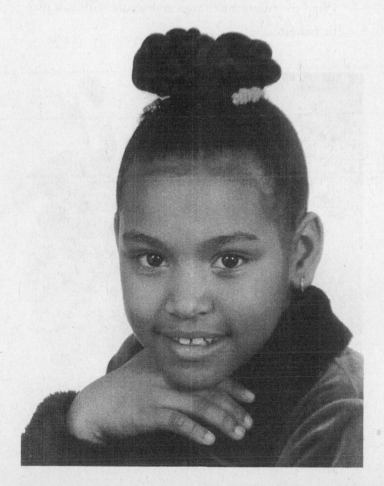

1. Gather the hair to the top of the head, and hold it firmly together at the crown with a soft hair band.

2. Separate the gathered hair into seven sections.

3. Make each section into a twist, so that there are seven twists.

4. Wrap the twists into a bun and secure with two plastic barrettes.

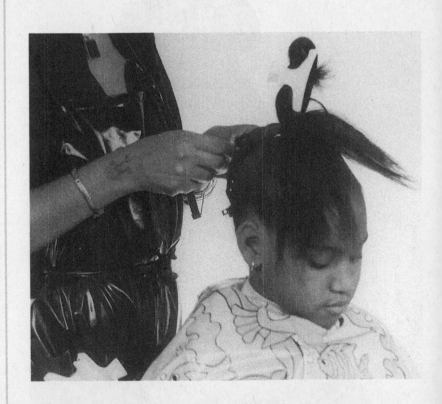

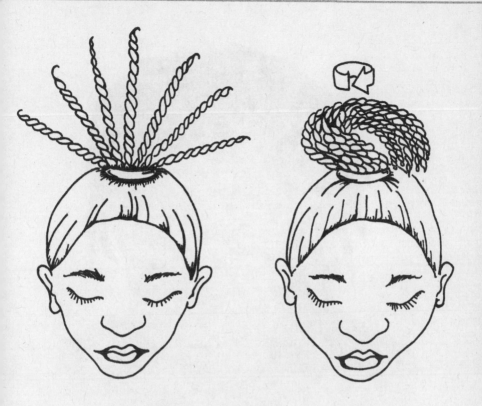

You can achieve different looks by twisting the hair flat to the head (similar to making a cornrow, which is explained in the next chapter) or into many twists, gathered up, hanging down, or a combination of the two. And the look will vary depending on if you style the hair when wet, after you blow-dry it, or after it dries naturally. You can also twist using an aloe vera–based gel on wet or dry hair.

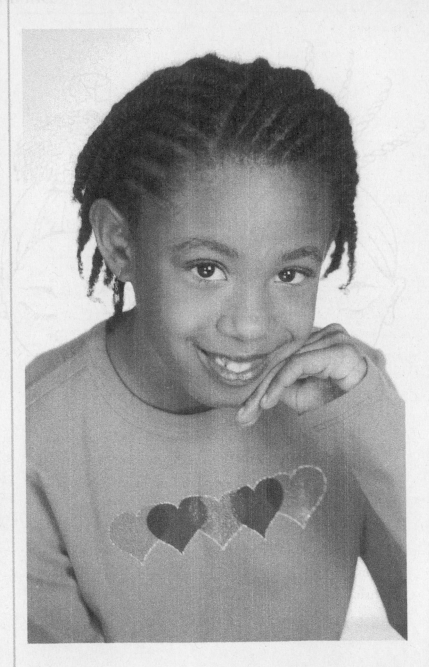

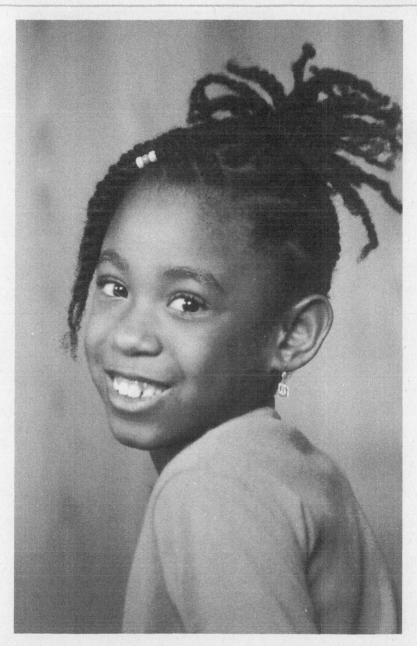

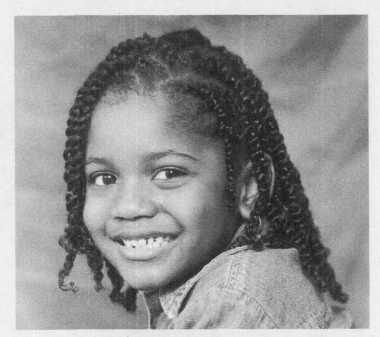

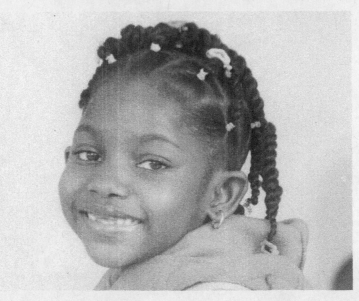

4

Twists, Cornrows, Zulu Knots, and Extensions

HAIR AFFIRMATIONS

Since I can remember, I've been aware (as are most Black women in our society) of the fascination with long, straight hair that so many of us suffer from. So I decided from the moment Jordan was born that I would do whatever I could to let her know that no matter how she styles her hair, no matter how her hair happens to look, she is much more than her hair, and that her beauty comes from within. Beginning before she was two, I started a ritual with her that we repeat to this day. Whenever we wash her hair, we stand in the full-length mirror after we've toweled it dry (before we have brushed or combed or braided it) and we do our chant: "I am BEAUTIFUL! I am SMART!" (And we reverse the order from time to time.) She always giggles and thinks it's pretty funny. But the cool thing is, now she does it with no prompting from me. I don't know what the long-term implications of our mantra will be—I certainly hope it helps to reinforce her sense of self-confidence. Right now, anyway, she does indeed think she is beautiful and smart!

—JOYE MERCER BARKSDALE

ow that you've learned how to do simple braids and twists, you're ready to move on to cornrows, double-strand flat twists, and zulu knots. Not only are these styles fashionable, but they can last up to two weeks, saving you hours of styling time.

Double-Stranded Flat Twists

1. Using a rat-tail comb, part the hair in six sections. The number of parts will vary with the hairstyle.

2. Starting at the hairline, grab two sections of hair of equal size—it's important here to make sure that the sections are equal or your twists will appear "lumpy."

3. Hold the hair between your thumb and index finger. Twist the right section over the left section and make an X.

4. Repeat this pattern three times. Before you make your fourth revolution, grab a section of hair from the right side equal to the two sections you hold in your hands.

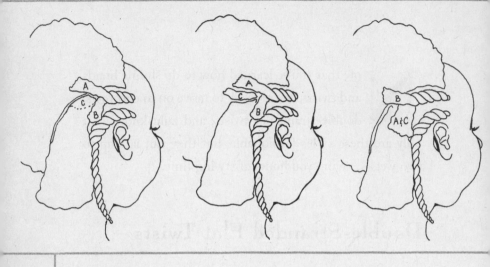

5. The right section should now be across your left between the index finger and your thumb. Your middle finger should now be holding the left section of hair, which is now on your right.

6. Bring the section of hair in your right hand over to the section of hair in your middle finger and now grasp both sections of hair with your right hand.

7. Now take the section of hair in your right hand and cross it over the section of hair in your left hand. Make an X with the two sections.

8. Repeat this pattern until you reach the bottom of the hair section.

Double-Stranded Twist with Ponytail

1. Blow-dry the hair.

2. Make eight parts from your child's forehead to the
   crown of her head.

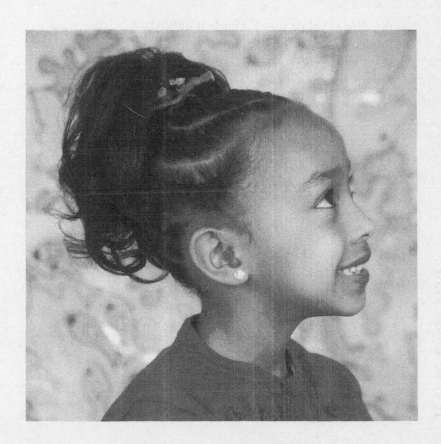

3. Use clips to section off hair. Attach a large clip to the hair at the top.

4. Twist the hair double-stranded until reaching the crown.

5. Twist a rubber band around the loose hair at top.

6. Use a curling iron for curls if desired.

You can also create hairstyles by combining double-stranded flat twists and two-stranded twists.

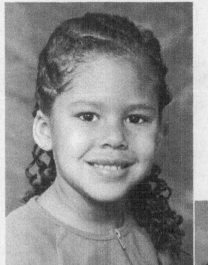

Double-Stranded Flat Twists with Stranded Twists Down the Back

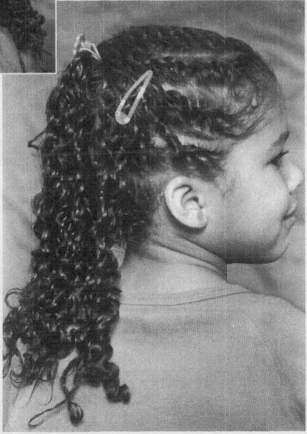

Double-Stranded Flat Twists with Two-Stranded Twists in the Back

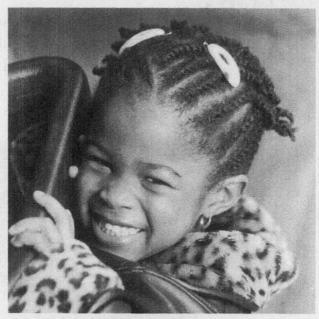

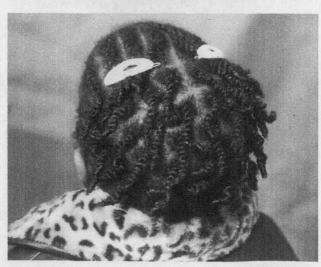

Double-Stranded Flat Twists in Two Ponytails

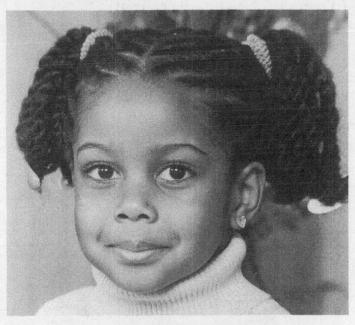

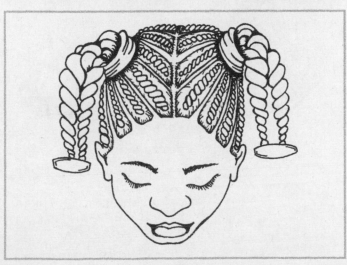

Flat Twists

Flat Twists with a Soft Fall

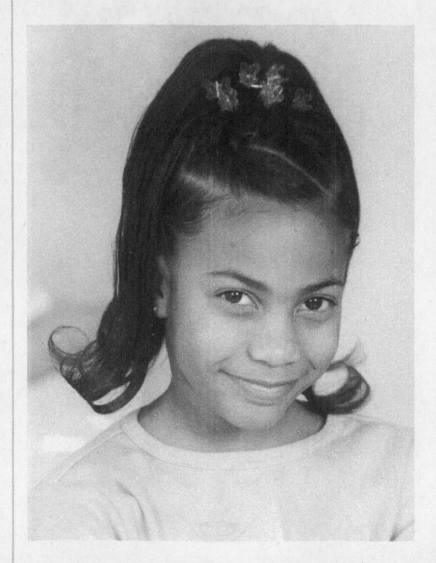

1. Part hair in the desired number of sections. (Here the hair is parted horizontally from ear to ear with a hair clip to section off the ponytail. It is also parted in a zig-zag style [see page 81 for instructions on zig-zag parts]).

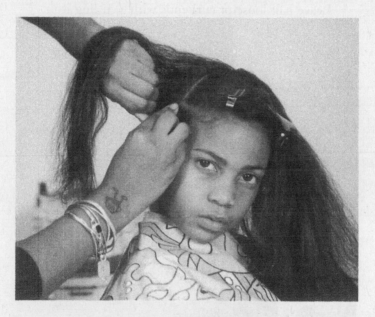

2. Take the desired section of hair and apply a small amount of water-based gel. Hold a section of hair with your right hand between your thumb and index finger.

3. With your right hand begin to roll-twist the hair between your thumb and index finger.

4. Then alternate and use your left hand to twist the hair. Continue this twisting pattern, until you reach the desired length of hair. Secure with a hair band. Leave hair loose or curl ends with a curling iron.

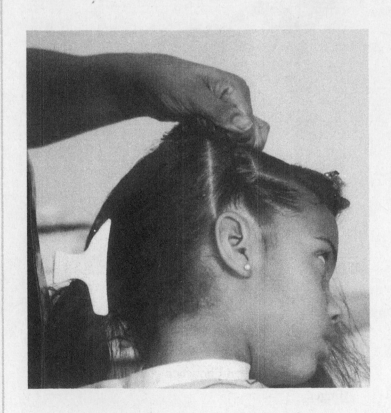

Connected Flat Twists with a Pulled-Up Ponytail

1. Using a rat-tail comb, make a half-circle parting for the bangs.

2. Again using the comb, make a whole circle parting around the head, using a hair clamp to section off hair for the ponytail.

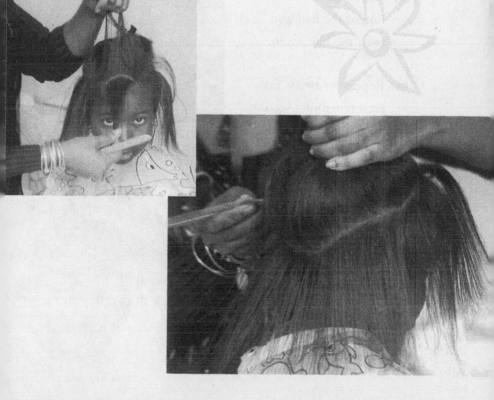

3. Part hair in each section into small squares.

4. Take the hair from one of these squares and use a small hair band to wrap around the hair. After securing the hair band, twist the hair until you reach the end.

5. Twist the hair into the adjoining section of hair. Wrap a rubber band around this section of the hair and twist the hair again.

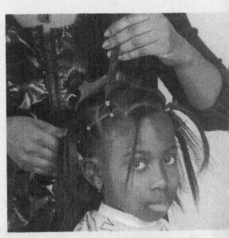

6. Repeat for twists for each remaining section of hair. When you have finished all the sections, gather all the loose hair into a ponytail and secure it with a clip.

7. Allow the hair to hang down loosely or curl with a curling iron if desired.

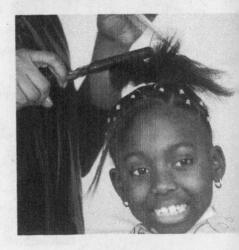

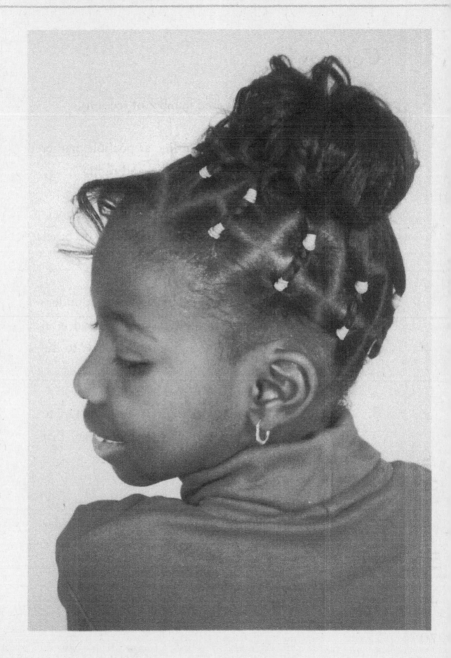

Cornrows

1. Part the hair in the desired number of sections.

2. Beginning as close to the hairline as possible, gather three sections of hair—left, middle, and right.

3. Hold the strand on the left side and cross it underneath the middle strand. The left strand now becomes the middle.

4. Now take the strand on your right and cross it underneath the middle strand. Now the right strand is in the middle. Repeat this pattern, going outside to the middle, three times.

5. As you begin the fourth revolution, you will start to pick up hair. On your left, grab a section of hair that is equal to the section of hair in your hand.

6. Bring this section and add it to the middle strand of the hair. Then continue to cross the left strand under the middle.

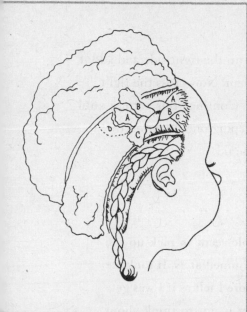

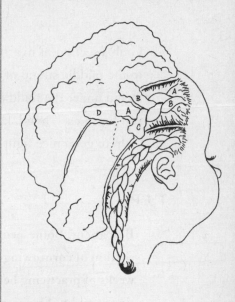

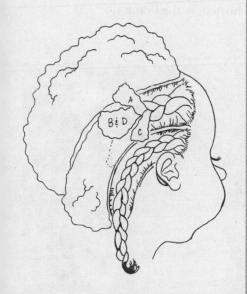

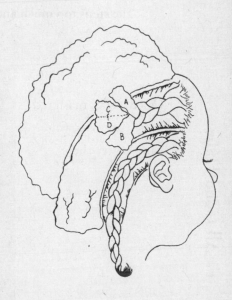

7. Grab a section of hair from the right side and add it to the middle strand of hair. Now cross the right strand under the middle. Continue this pattern until you finish each braid, keeping one finger on the scalp to get a nice tight braid.

TIP . . . .

> Be patient. Some people seem to pick up the rhythm of cornrowing immediately. It took me weeks of practicing before I felt as if I was getting it right. The secret is not to think about the steps too much and just enjoy the braiding.

Once you've mastered basic cornrows, you can also try these variations:

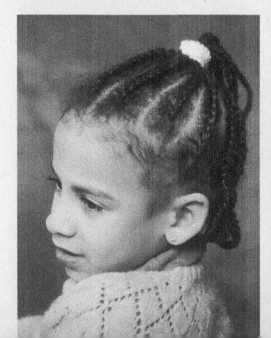

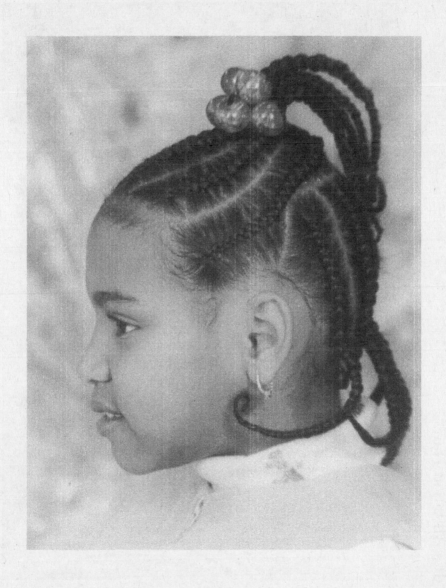

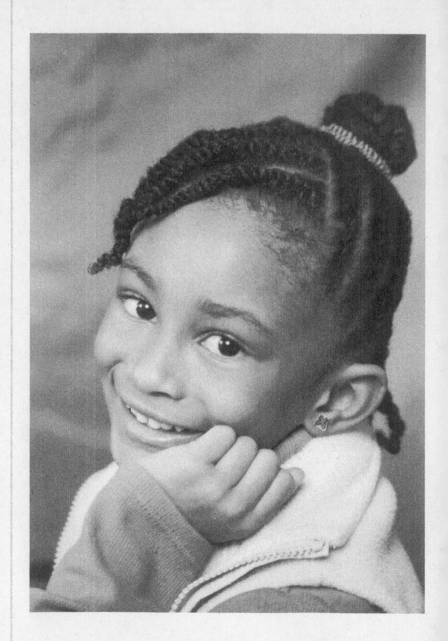

TWISTS AND BRAIDS MAINTENANCE

Twists and cornrows are wonderful hairstyles and can be worn for up to two weeks. To keep your child's cornrows and twists looking neat, tie a scarf around your child's head before he or she goes to bed at night.

Sometimes you may need to retwist or rebraid some of the twists or cornrows that have come loose.

TAKING OUT TWISTS AND BRAIDS

Try to take out twists and cornrows every two weeks. If you let the hairstyle stay in longer, your child's hair may begin to lock, and it will be difficult and painful to take the twists and cornrows out.

Don't try to take out the twists or cornrows all at once or you'll end up with a head full of tangled hair. Instead, take out each cornrow individually and comb through that section of hair. Use a clip to separate the hair that you have already untwisted, so it won't get tangled after you comb it.

Use your fingers or the end of the rat-tail comb. Start at the end of the twist or cornrow and gently begin to untwist the hair. Don't be tempted to start in the middle of the braid or twists because you think it will be faster; it isn't. Your child will just start complaining that it hurts too much.

Zulu, Bantu, or Nubian Knots

1. Section the hair into squares or triangles. Make the parts as big or as small as you want. Divide the hair in the first section into two equal sections.

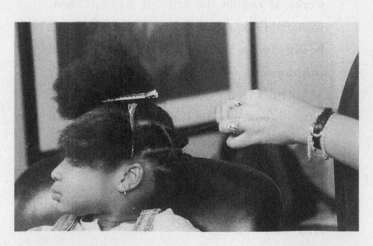

2. Using a nonflaking gel, twist the hair into two-strand twists.

3. Once you have finished twisting the hair, hold the hair at the end. Placing your index finger on the scalp, begin to twist the hair into a ball or knot shape.

4. Tuck the end of the hair under the knot you have just created.

5. Repeat until all sections are done.

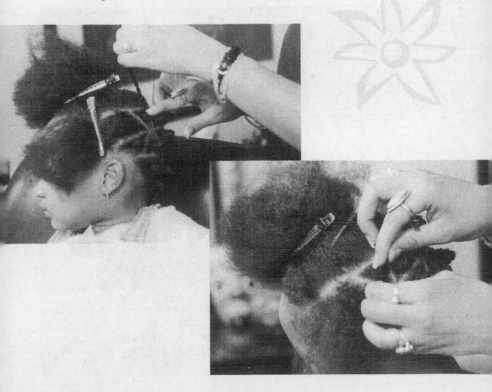

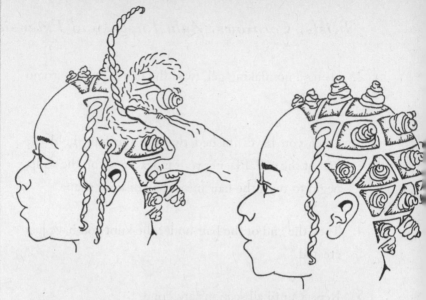

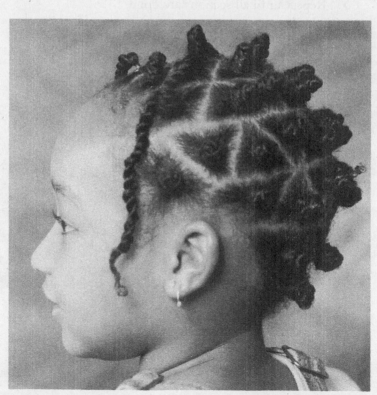

Zulu Knots

Here the knots were styled in a similar fashion except the hair was blow-dried before it was styled. To finish the style, butterfly clips were used as an accent.

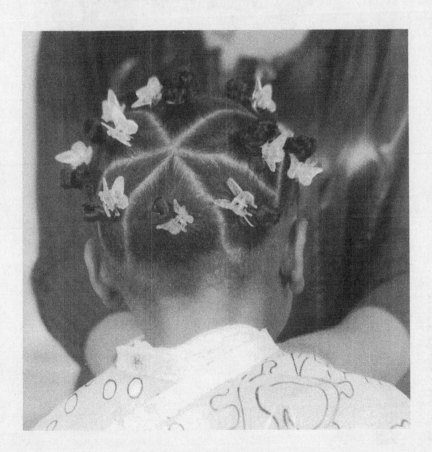

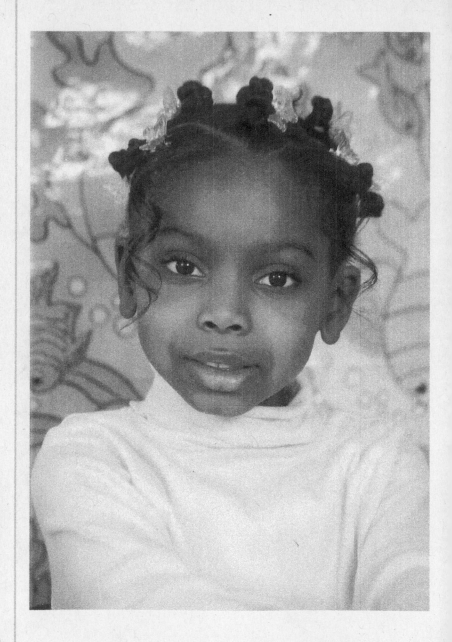

Zig-Zag Parts

I f you want to put some flair into your styles, start using zig-zag parts instead of straight parts. Don't be afraid. If you can draw a zig-zag, you will be able to do these parts.

1. Take the end of the rat-tooth comb and place the comb at the point where you would like the part to begin. Gently use the comb to make a line in the hair as shown.

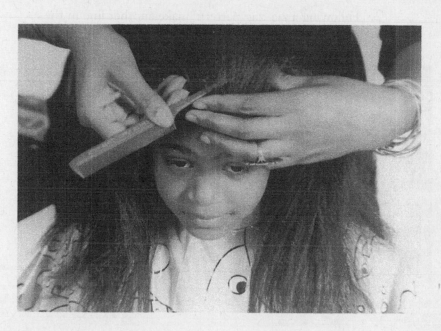

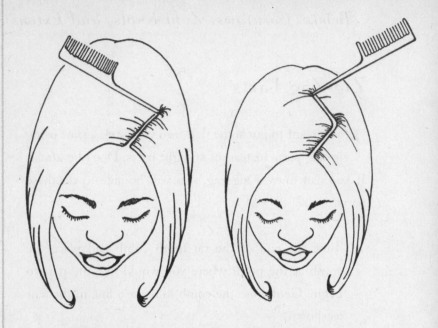

2. Following a zig-zag pattern, make another line in the
   hair as shown.

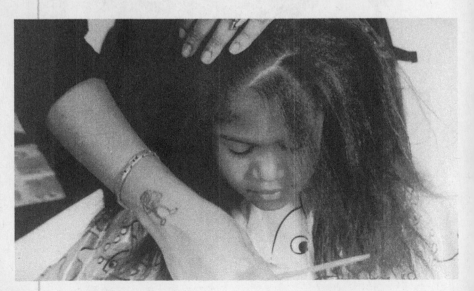

3. Continue parting and separating the hair until you complete the pattern you want. Once you've mastered this, you can make the zig-zags as small or as large as you want.

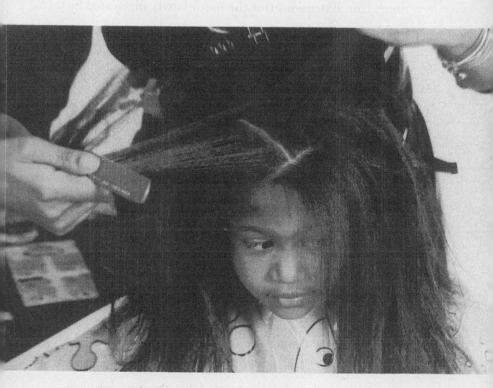

Extensions

This book won't focus too much on extensions because the average parent can't put extensions in their children's hair. Extensions (for the uninitiated) are created by braiding or weaving hair (synthetic or human) into a person's hair to create various hairstyles. Go to a professional braider to get an attractive, properly styled braiding job like the one shown here.

Here are some things to think about when considering extensions for your child's hair:

- Resist the temptation to put extensions in little girls' hair. I see countless girls as young as three years old with braid extensions down their backs. The hair is too heavy for their heads and will almost certainly cause hair breakage. Try one of the attractive styles in this book instead.

- Little girls cannot sit still long enough for braid extensions. Most adults have a hard enough time sitting in a chair for six hours for a braiding job. Just think about what torture this can be for a child.

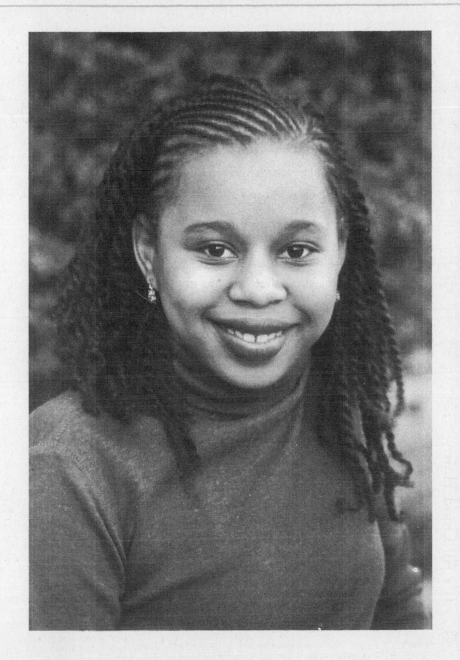

- If you do decide to get extensions for your child, don't skimp on the hair. When you or your child decides it is the right time to put extensions in their hair, don't be cheap. Spend money on some quality hair, like the Kanekalon brand. Cheap hair can cause scalp irritation. Think about how upset you will be when you have to take your child's hair out after three days because she can't stop scratching her scalp.

- If your child says the braids are too tight, believe her. If your child's hair is braided properly, she should not be complaining that it is too tight or that it hurts. Don't believe anyone who suggests that the pain will wear off in a few days. Braids that are too tight can lead to hair breakage and, eventually, hair loss.

- Take the braids out after three months (or the length of time suggested by your stylist). It may be tempting to let your child sport that hairdo for a few weeks longer, but you will definitely be sorry when you go to take it out. Your child's hair will start to lock, and it will be *very* painful to take the extensions out.

5 Swimmer's Hair

NOT FRIZZY OR NAPPY, BUT BEAUTIFUL

A lot of mothers of Biracial children don't know what to do with their children's hair. That's why you see a lot of Biracial children with hair that looks really dry and as if it hadn't been done in four or five days. I was determined that my daughter wasn't going to look like that.

I grew up in a predominantly Black neighborhood, and I was always doing my girlfriends' hair. So I knew how to do Black hair. But Whitney has this middle-of-the-road hair between White and Black hair. So it's tough to find products that work on her hair. The Black products are too heavy and the White products don't do anything for her hair. I keep saying I'm going to develop some products for interracial girls. For a while, Whitney asked me to buy White products for frizzy hair. I told her, "Girl, you don't have frizzy hair. You have nappy hair."

Whitney has a lot of White friends, so she went through this whole phase where she hated her hair. Her friends have hair that they can brush, blow-dry, and go. She would say, "I wish my hair was straight, and my edges are so nappy."

But I think she's made peace with her hair now. One of teachers told her, "Whitney, I see you with so many different hairstyles. You can do anything with your hair." I hope she realizes that.

—LINDA TURBERT

There's no need to cry the summertime blues anymore just because your kids are headed to the swimming pool and you don't want to deal with that wet hair. Many of the twists and cornrow styles featured below and elsewhere in the book will free you from having to style your children's hair every time they go to the pool or to the beach.

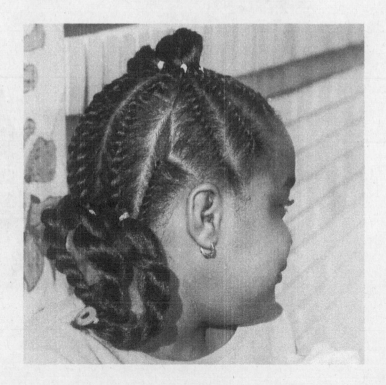

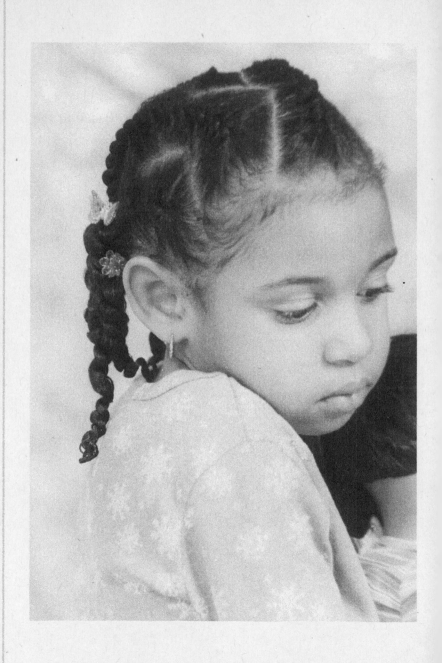

Cornrow and twist styles are perfect for swimming and can be worn for up to two weeks. Here are some tips:

- Put a swim cap on your child's hair to provide protection from the chlorine.

- When your child gets out of the water, rinse the twists or cornrows really well to remove the chlorine or saltwater.

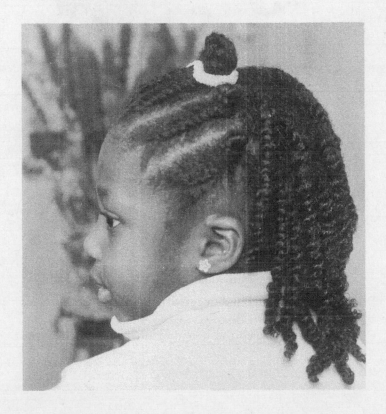

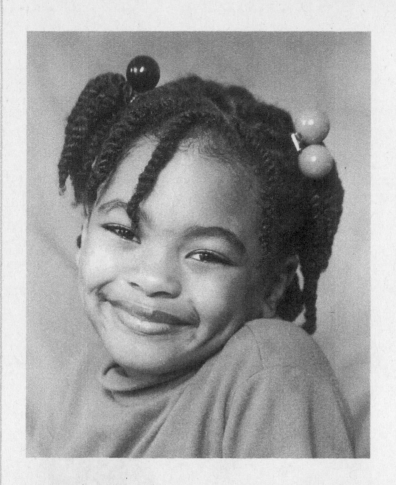

- If any of the individual twists or cornrows comes loose, simply rebraid or retwist them.

- Be sure you keep the hair moisturized by using hair oil.

6 Locks

A LIFE-CHANGING STYLE

Locks have changed my relationship with my daughter Aja. Before she got locks, I had a time with her hair. It was so thick and tangly. I had to go through so much to wash it and comb it.

I'd try to be gentle, but she'd cry. I was so frustrated. I'd take her to salons, but after they did her hair they would tell me not to bring her back because her hair was so thick and she was so tender-headed. Once she even threw up in a stylist's lap.

It got so bad, I'd have my husband, Warren, take her because the stylists would feel sorry for him and do her hair because they thought he couldn't do it.

Finally, when Aja was ten, she decided she wanted to lock her hair. Warren was against it because he said folks treated him differently because of his locks. Security people follow him in stores, and the police stop him all the time. He didn't want people to see her hair and put her in a category.

But I went to him and said, "We've given our children the skills to make decisions for themselves. It's her hair, let her make the decision." Aja had done all her research; she had talked to people with locks and decided this is what she wanted to do. The best thing about locks, she says, is that you do not have to comb your hair. The only thing she said was that she didn't want any big "do-do locks."

Now I don't have to do hair. Aja's sister, Ife, also has locks and they do their hair themselves. They twist it, braid it, tie it up, put crinkles in it, and I am a happy woman. I can truly say that locks have improved my relationship with my daughters.

—SHARON ADAMS-TAYLOR

To Lock or Not to Lock

Although your child may have just discovered locks, Africans have been wearing the hairstyle for centuries. Today, African-Americans are returning to locks as a symbol of pride and embracing the texture of their kinky hair.

Some children want to wear locks to make a statement about their African heritage. Others are simply tired of braiding or curling their hair and want a low-maintenance hairstyle. Others want more length. Locking the hair encourages tightly curled hair to grow. When you lock hair, you pretty much leave it alone. You don't comb or brush it, relax it or hot curl it, all of which can cause hair breakage. After about six months to a year, the hair is said to be locked.

Locks are not for every child. The hairstyle is permanent. If your daughter or son is the type who wants a new hairstyle every couple of months, tell her or him to try a different style. If your child has doubts, encourage her or him to wear the comb twists or coils. If your child decides not to lock, she or he can take the twists or coils out before the hair begins to lock. If your child wants a different hairstyle after the hair locks, the locks will have to be cut off.

Locks are recommended for children who are confident and can talk about their hair choices. A lot of people don't understand locks and may say cruel things to children about their hairstyle. When his friends start to call him "Buckwheat," he may decide he doesn't want locks. Moreover, the transition time between when locks are started and when the hair actually locks can be rough if

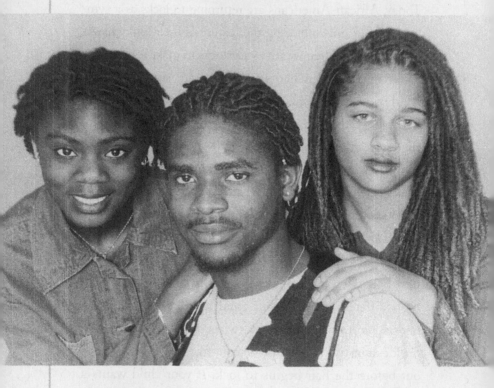

your child is not used to wearing a natural hairstyle. Talk to your child about the locking process and have him talk to other people who wear the hairstyle.

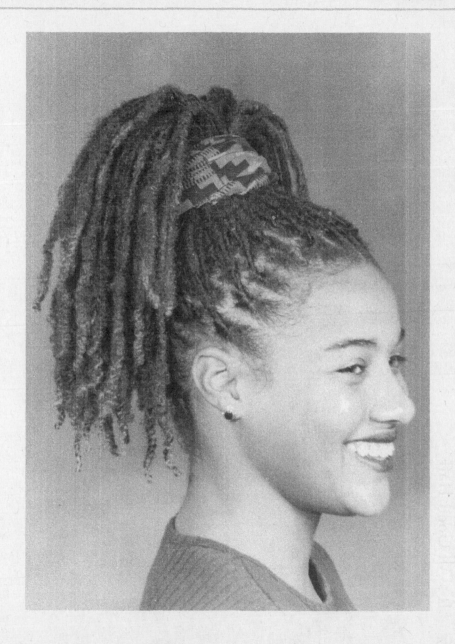

Locking can only be done on natural hair. Your child has two options if her hair has been chemically straightened. She can choose to cut her hair and start the locking process. However, most girls say they would prefer to let their relaxers grow out; that is, let new virgin hair grow to a length where they can feel comfortable cutting the relaxed hair off.

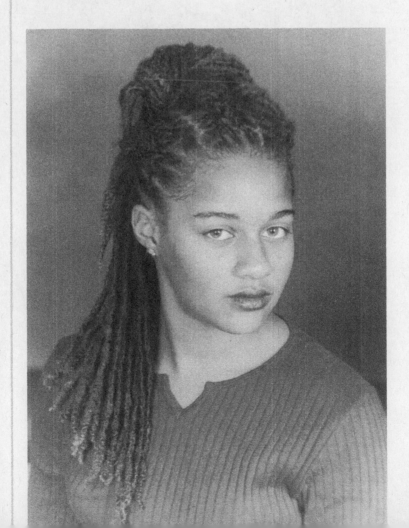

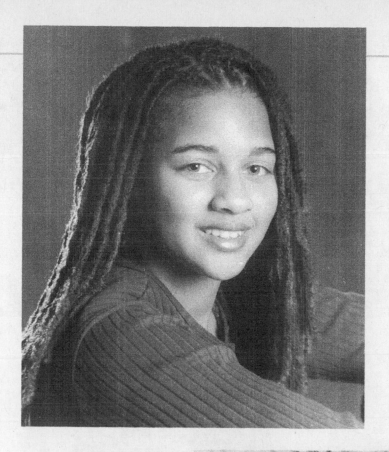

Your daughter or son has lots of styling options with locks. They can be worn up or down. If you braid them after shampooing, and remove the braids, the locks will have a crinkly look.

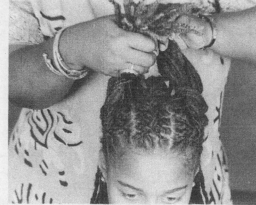

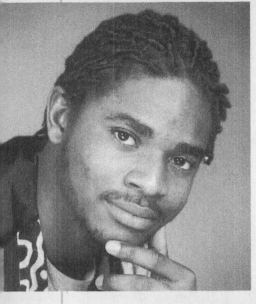

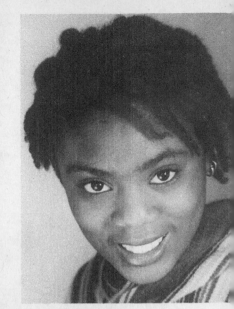

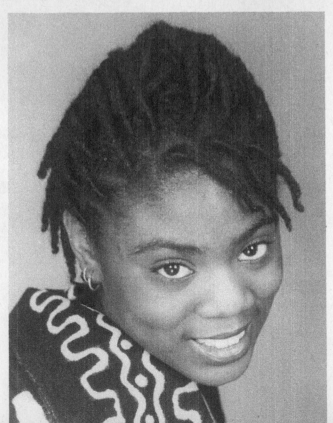

Misconceptions About Locks

It's just a whole bunch of nappy, dirty hair.

Locks are formed by hair meshing or locking together. Locks that are properly groomed are beautiful and can be styled in a variety of gorgeous styles.

People who wear locks don't wash their hair.

People who wear locks wash their hair just as the rest of us do.

Dreadlocks is the name for locks.

Don't refer to locks as "dreadlocks": There is nothing *dreadful* about locks.

Using beeswax will help the hair lock better.

A water-based gel is a better choice for locking hair. Beeswax will cause the hair to mat and get dirty.

How to Lock Hair

To get beautifully styled locks, I would recommend getting them started by a professional stylist. Don't just pick the first stylist who says they can lock hair. If you know people with locks you admire, ask them where they got their hair done. Ask for a consultation at the salon and ask if the stylist has locked children's hair before.

However, if you feel confident that you can lock hair, by all means, use the following directions.

Palm-Rolling

1. Using a rat-tail comb on clean wet hair, part the entire head, horizontally, starting from the hairline and going to the nape.

2. Divide the hair into subparts from the right side of the hair to the left. Make these parts as big or as small as you want. If you want larger locks, make bigger parts. If you want smaller locks, make smaller parts.

3. Hold the section of hair in your left hand. Using the tip of your right hand, roll the hair in one complete motion.

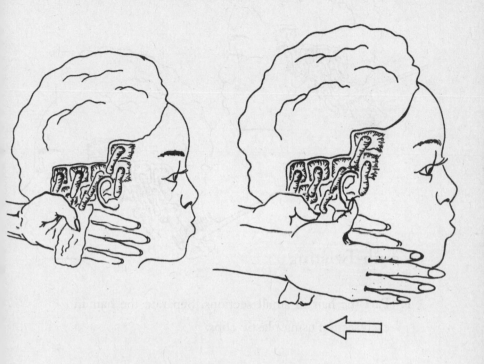

4. Place a metal clip on each lock to help it stay in place as you lock the hair.

5. Repeat these steps until you have locked the entire head.

6. Place your child under the dryer until her hair is dry.

7. Remove the clips.

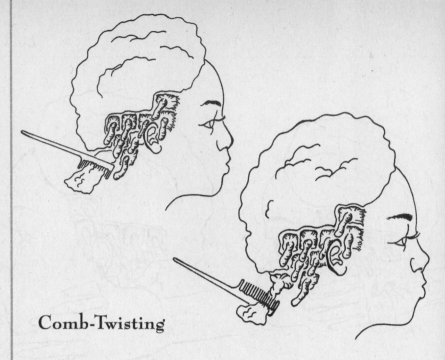

Comb-Twisting

1. Part the hair in small sections. Separate the hair in each section using plastic clips.

2. Starting at the nape of the neck, place a small amount of water-based gel on a section of hair.

3. Using a rat-tail comb, place the comb at the end of a section of hair and twist the hair around the comb until it forms a coil.

4. Place a metal or plastic clip on each coil until you finish twisting the entire head.

5. Place your child under the dryer.

TIP . . . .

Comb twists have become a popular hairstyle for natural hair. Your child can still wear this hairstyle even if she doesn't want to lock her hair.

WASHING AND MAINTAINING LOCKS

Forget about the instructions to put Sea Breeze and Witch Hazel on your child's scalp to keep it clean when you are first locking hair.

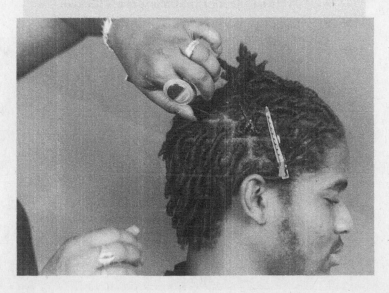

Children's hair gets dirty, and you need to wash it on a regular basis. You want to wash the hair as gently as possible so you disturb as few coils as possible. Start by using your fingertips to wash the scalp. Then use shampoo to clean the locks, being careful not to scrub. Rinse the head. Make sure you remove all traces of dirt and lint. Condition the hair. After shampooing the hair, you will need to retwist all the coils that have come loose.

Every few weeks, you will need to retwist your locks as they grow. Twisting is necessary to get the new virgin hair growing in to lock and to retwist the hair that has already locked.

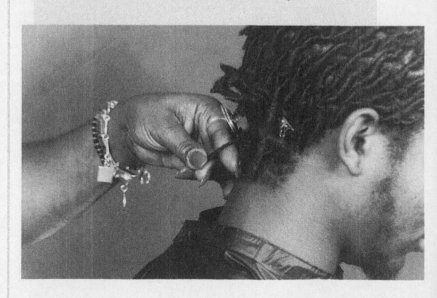

7 How to Relax Hair

"SALON" WOES

When my youngest daughter, Coco, was about ten or eleven years old, she really liked the way her best friend Cajun's hair looked. Cajun, who was Biracial and had, let's just say, a different grade of hair than Coco, suggested that Coco get her hair done by Cajun's auntie, who was a hairstylist and always did Cajun's hair.

I told Coco that her hair was never going to

look like Cajun's because she had a different texture hair. But Coco said she'd really wanted her hair to look like Cajun's. Anyway, I dropped Coco off for her ten o'clock appointment and went off to run errands. When I got back to pick her up at noon, I walked into a scene that would have been funny if Coco hadn't looked so sad. Here was the auntie, madly working on Coco's hair, which looked like a blown-out greasy Afro—and not a curl in sight—trying to get it to look like a style someone other than the bride of Frankenstein would wear.

When I walked in, the auntie said, "It'll curl, it'll curl. We just gotta let it set for a day or two then she'll really like it." Though I had my doubts, I paid her. She said to bring Coco back in a few days if the curl didn't "show up." It didn't.

I took her back and waited while the auntie worked on it some more. Finally, she rolled it in some perm rods and let it sit for a while.

When she took them out, there were some bends in some of the hair strands, but nothing like the Jheri curls I'd seen folks wear. We decided to give up.

When Coco went to school, the kids teased her unmercifully, calling her Afrobaby and worse. She came home in tears. After a couple of weeks, my sister told me that her friend had had the same problem, and that she'd gotten hers fixed beautifully by a hairstylist not far away. I agreed to try.

Well, I'm not sure what this lady did, but I think she put in a relaxer, even though she'd been told that another chemical had been used a couple of weeks before. Anyway, when I picked up Coco, she looked really cute.

BUT—a week later, her hair started falling out! I mean, this child's hair was getting thinner and thinner, and at some places, there was just a bit of thick peach fuzz on her scalp!

I ended up taking her to my hairstylist who, for a substantially higher price, cut Coco's hair attractively, and she wore it in a short little cute style. Over the next weeks, my stylist conditioned it and took care of it until it grew back. Needless to say, we've never been back to "auntie" or to the fix-it woman.

—KAREN DAVIS

109

About Relaxing Hair

You've all seen the pretty pictures of the little girls on the perm boxes with the beautiful, bouncy hair. Lately, you've been thinking that relaxing your child's hair would make your life much easier because you wouldn't have to spend so much time managing and styling it. Or, maybe it's your daughter—or even your son—who's pushing for the change.

Thousands of mothers are successful at relaxing their children's hair. Relaxers can make your child's hair easier to comb and style. Nor do you have to worry about your child swelling up that hairstyle you spent hours creating with the straightening comb. Permanent waves and permanent creme relaxers, however, are chemicals that can also damage the hair. So you need to keep the following in mind: Permanent waves put curl in the hair; permanent creme relaxers straighten the hair. However, they are both chemicals.

Let a professional relax your child's hair, especially if you don't have experience applying relaxers. The money you save from doing it yourself is not worth it if you damage your child's hair. The money and time you would spend to help her grow back a healthy head of hair could be astronomical—and a huge burden on you and your child!

Wait until she is at least eight years old to relax your child's hair. Because most children's hair texture can change several times as they grow, stylists say their hair does not generally mature until they are at least eight years old. But, as stylist Jill Carpenter puts it, if "it is clear that the mother is going to put a relaxer in the child's hair, I would rather put it in than have the mother do it and damage the child's hair."

Never use a relaxer on your child's hair if it is broken or if her scalp is irritated. Relaxing damaged hair will just cause hair to break off. If there are sores on your child's scalp, the relaxer will cause the scalp to burn.

Don't leave the relaxer on too long. Most of us remember the relaxer dance we did as little girls. As your mother applied the relaxer to your hair, she took a little too long. Then your scalp started to tingle and you started to fidget in the chair. Then your mother said, "Girl, sit still. It doesn't hurt that bad, and I still need to work the rest of this relaxer in." Meanwhile, your scalp was on fire!

"So many parents will say, 'This child's hair is so nappy, I think I'll leave it on a little longer so it will get straighter,'" says dermatologist Dr. Valerie Callender. Don't be tempted to leave the relaxer on longer than what is stated on the manufacturer's directions. Leaving it on the child's head will only damage the child's hair and will cause her scalp to burn and leave scabs.

Apply the relaxer only to your child's new growth. When doing a retouch, be careful not to overlap with hair that has already been chemically relaxed. If you do, you will certainly damage the hair.

Wait six to eight weeks before touchups. The manufacturers aren't crazy. Your child's hair doesn't need a touchup every three to four weeks just because her hair isn't as straight as you would like it to be. Touchups that are too frequent will also lead to hair breakage and scalp irritation.

Use the appropriate relaxer for your child's hair. Relaxers generally come in three strengths—mild, medium, and super. Do not assume that because your daughter's hair is "really kinky" that you need the super-strength. If you are not sure what strength to use, let a stylist put the relaxer in your daughter's hair.

Relaxers need regular maintenance. Don't think that once you relax your child's hair that you're done. She must get regular touchups to keep her hair looking healthy. We all have heard jokes about children who desperately need their hair retouched. But there is nothing funny about the hair breakage that can result from waiting too long between relaxer retouches.

Hair breakage occurs because the point on the hair where the new growth and the relaxer meet is very weak. The daily combing and brushing of the hair can cause the hair to become damaged and break. As a parent, you need to commit to relaxing hair. If you don't want to relax the hair anymore, braid your child's hair to eliminate having to constantly comb or brush it. Or, let your child's hair grow out until it gets long enough that you can cut the relaxer out.

No-lye relaxers and kiddie relaxers can still damage hair. Parents assume that some relaxers that contain lye are too harsh for their daughter's hair. Or mothers assume that because they are using a kiddie relaxer, the relaxer is milder. No-lye and kiddie relaxers still contain a straightening ingredient that can damage your child's hair.

How to Properly Relax Your Child's Hair

Before you get started, you need to have these items on hand:

Gloves

Base (oil, petroleum jelly, hair or scalp grease)

Relaxer

Rat-tail comb or tint brush

Neutralizing shampoo

Conditioner

Wide-tooth comb

TIP . . . .

Try to make sure your daughter does not scratch her scalp before you put a relaxer in her hair because it could cause her scalp to burn. Also, if she has had her hair braided, try to wait a week before you relax her hair because the perm could also damage her scalp.

Note: The following instructions are for putting a relaxer in virgin hair (hair without any type of chemicals).

1. Part the hair in four sections. Make a center part from the front of the forehead to the nape of the neck. And from ear to ear. Use clamps to section off the hair.

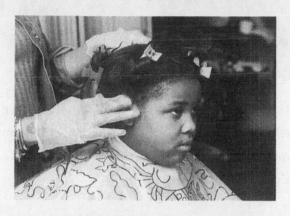

2. Using a comb, make half-inch partings. Using your gloved fingers, apply relaxer base to your child's entire scalp and forehead.

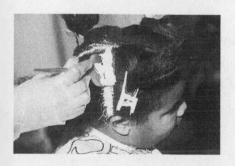
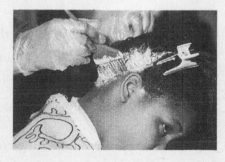

3. Starting at the scalp, apply relaxer using the rat-tail comb or tint brush to the ends of the hair.

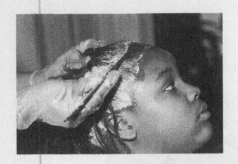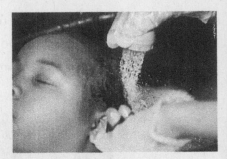

4. Use the tips of your fingers to smooth the relaxer. The relaxer should stay on the hair no longer than twenty minutes. If the relaxer starts to burn your child's hair, rinse it out immediately.

5. After relaxing the hair, rinse it thoroughly with warm water. Make sure you rinse out all the relaxer, especially at the nape of the neck because it is the most difficult area to rinse.

6. After rinsing the hair thoroughly, shampoo the hair with a neutralizing shampoo. Don't forget the neck, forehead, and the nape of the neck. Rinse and shampoo two more times.

7. Apply a moisturizing conditioner and place a plastic cap on your child's hair. Place your child under the dryer for ten to fifteen minutes.

8. Rinse the hair again after your child comes from under the dryer, then apply a styling solution—a mousse or a setting lotion that will help protect the hair from the heat of the blow-dryer—and gently dry again.

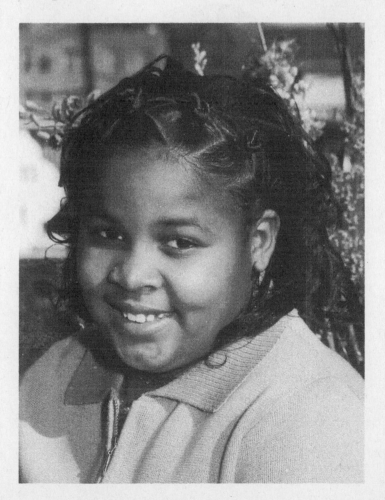

For more information on relaxed hair, go to the Web site www.blackkidshair.com.

Here's another style that's perfect for relaxed hair.

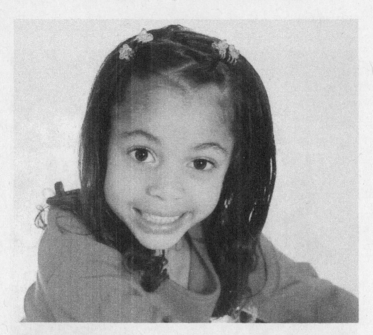

My daughter Maya's hair does not have a relaxer in it, but the style would easily work on relaxed or pressed (straightened with a straightening comb) hair.

Here, the hair was lightly pressed and then zig-zag parts were added in the front of Maya's hair. Then two flat twists in the front and the ends were styled with a curling iron.

8 How to Blow-Dry Hair

"HAIRDUE"

When I found out that Ari was going to be a girl, I was thrilled. But the next thing I thought about was the hair. What would I do? Would I develop the magical power to do hair once they delivered her into my arms?

I had never done my own hair. I cut it off or braided it. I reasoned I had time to decide before she was born. Most kids were born bald or nearly bald. But of course when Ari was delivered into my arms, she had a full head of hair. "Isn't this abnormal?" I asked the nurse. "It's great, isn't it?" said the nurse. "I don't think so," I must have muttered under my breath. Well, at least all I had to do was brush it.

By the time she was ten months old, though her hair had thickened and multiplied, I had considered locks for Ari, but felt that she should make the choice about what to do with her hair. But that was before the day came when I spent three hours trying to coax Ari into a 'do and she screamed as if she was on fire. That day I made the decision: it was locks or bust.

I started her locks in New York. People have always thought I was making a political statement with my short hair or braids. I was always making a practical one, which is what happened with Ari. When she turned six, she wanted the locks out because the kids teased her, she said. Ari wanted to be more "normal." I cut off her beautiful shoulder-length locks and showed Ari her reflection in the mirror. One tear trickled down her cheek. "Can you put them back?" she asked.

No, I told her, as I wiped her cheek dry, but I promised her that the next day we would get it braided. We set off to the stylist who did a fabulous job, and Ari was happy with her braids for three years. Recently, I suggested she put her locks back in and she did this year. Who knows what Ari's path will finally be? But I know I've set one tone—low maintenance.

—VASHTI DUBOIS

Blow-Drying Your Child's Hair

Sometimes you may want to blow-dry your child's hair for a different look. You may also find that the blow-dryer makes it easier for you to comb your child's hair. Blow-drying loosens the curl pattern of the hair, making it softer and longer. Just be careful not to blow hot hair onto the scalp because you could burn your child's head.

1. Separate the hair into several sections and use clamps to keep it separate.

2. Use a blow-drying lotion to help protect the hair.

3. You can blow-dry with a brush or a comb attachment. If you're like me, you may find it's easier to use the plastic comb attachment. With the brush in one hand, start brushing the ends of one of the sections of hair.

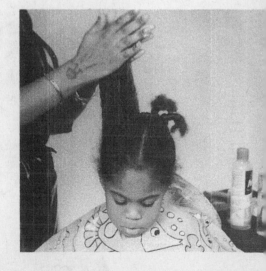

4. With the blow-dryer in the other hand, use the nozzle to blow air on the hair. Continue working your way down the shaft of the hair, using the brush and the blow-dryer until you reach the scalp.

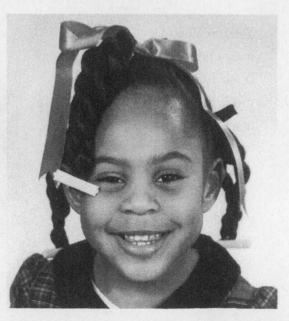

5. If you use the comb attachment, place the comb attachment on the ends of one section of hair and begin to comb the hair to the ends. Continue combing your way down the shaft of the hair, until you reach the scalp.

9 Boys' Hair

OLD WIVES' TALES

There are lots of old wives' tales about cutting Black people's hair. They tell you not to cut little boys' hair until they turn two because it will slow their speech. Then there's the other one that says you should cut the hair on the full moon, because it will grow back quicker and fuller.

I cut my first son's hair when he was one, and he has to go to a speech therapist now. You don't know if there is anything to that old wives' tale, but it kind of makes you go *hmmmm.*

We haven't cut James's hair yet and he is two and a half. I'm kind of going with the flow, because in Jimmy's family a lot of men have long hair, so it's kind of a family tradition. James really likes to get his hair cornrowed. He'll come sit in my lap and say, "Mommy, plait my hair."

—CARLA CROMER-BUTLER

Boys and the Barbershop

When my son, Michael, was born, every Black woman I know told me not to cut his hair before he turned two years old. Terrible things would happen, they warned, if I dared to cut his hair. He wouldn't learn to talk when he was supposed to. His hair would turn nappy or he would be short. These old wives' tales have been around for generations. Do I believe in old wives' tales? No. Was I going to tempt fate by cutting my son's hair? . . . I let that child's hair grow until he was two years old!

By the time he was two, though, I was tired of running after my son to try to brush his little Afro. So off I headed to the local barbershop. I wasn't really up on my barbershop lingo, but I explained that I wanted some taken off the top and shorter on the sides. The barber nodded, took the clippers, and proceeded to take all my baby's hair off. Later my husband laughed at his son's skinned head and told me most barbers didn't like to cut little boys' heads.

Luckily, I found someone who did like to cut little kids' heads. She's a sister named Billye, and she works as a stylist at a children's hair salon called Cartoon Cuts. She cuts Michael's hair exactly the way my husband and I want it, and now Michael won't let anyone else cut his hair.

My friends have their own stories of taking their son from barber to barber until they find one who is patient enough to cut boys' hair. Single moms say barbershops are intimidating. It can be tough to walk into a barbershop full of men and not know enough of the language to explain how to get your son's hair cut.

Here are some suggestions and terms to make your next trip to the barbershop more successful:

- Ask other parents for recommendations for barbers who enjoy cutting boys' heads. Many barbers are just not patient enough to cut little boys' heads. Boys fidget, move their heads, and cry. As a result, many barbers would just as soon not cut your sons' hair. Ask your friends who cuts their sons' hair.

- When you find a barber, watch him cut some boys' heads. Is he or she patient? Does he talk to your son? Is he in a hurry or is he trying to make sure he does a good job? Is the haircut even, or does the barber leave uneven patches of hair? Does he explain his tools and what he uses them for?

• Make sure the shop is clean and is a place where you and your son are comfortable. Make sure that the barbers clean their tools. Listen in on their conversations. If you don't want your son listening to a lot of swearing and grown-folks conversations, find another barbershop.

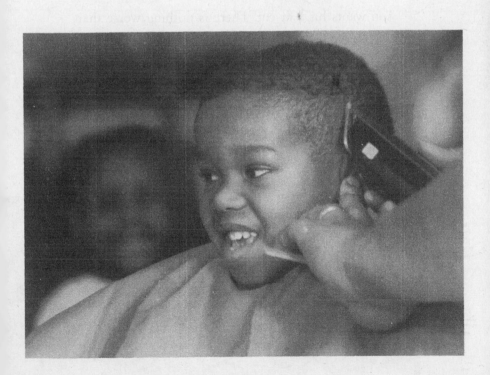

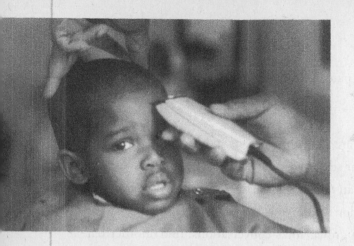

• Make sure the barber understands how you or your son wants his hair cut. There is nothing worse than asking the barber to take a little off the top and then seeing him take the clippers and mow almost all his hair off. A good barber will take time to understand exactly how you want your son's hair cut. A good barber will cut it a little longer than you want and then ask you if would like the hair to be cut shorter.

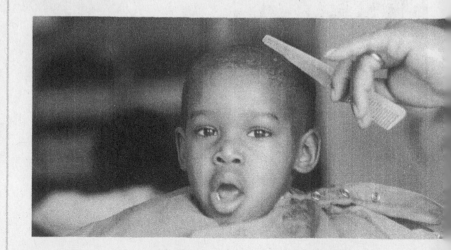

Here are some popular haircuts for boys. The barber used a clipper with a guard to cut and shape the hair. The size of the guard determines how close the hair will be cut.

The Fade

Hair is cut short on top and close on the sides.

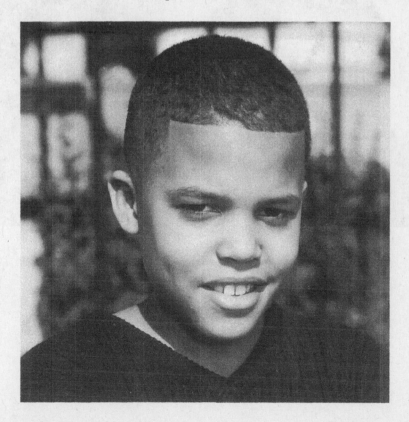

The All Even

Hair is cut even all around the head. Wash hair once a week; use a light oil and brush.

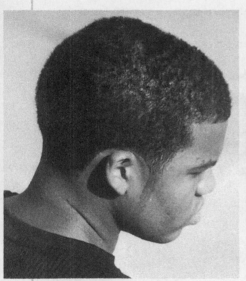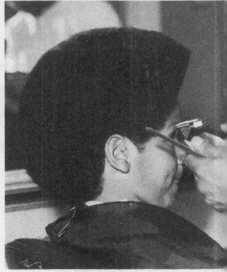

The Afro

Hair is allowed to grow out several inches. That 1970s big Afro has recently made a comeback. But parents still have the same old complaint: The hair doesn't look neat. To make sure an Afro stays well groomed, follow these tips:

- Buy your son a pick to comb his hair. Make sure he combs the hair from the root to the ends. If he doesn't comb his hair every day, it will become matted and very difficult to comb.

- Consider braiding his hair in cornrows at night so his hair will stay neater and will be easier to comb.

- Wash the hair often so it will stay clean.

- Take your son to the barber for a shape-up every three weeks. A well-groomed Afro is easier to comb.

- Keep the hair moisturized with hair oil.

Twists and Cornrows

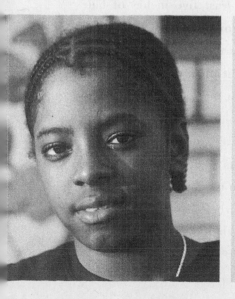 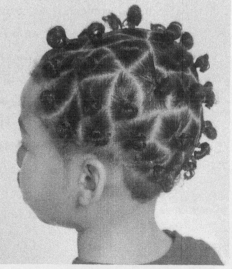

Inspired by their basketball and rap heroes, boys are wearing cornrows and twists, too.

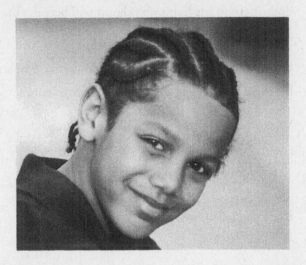

TIP . . . .

Stylists say you need at least five inches of hair before you can wear cornrows or twists. It can take from four to eight months to grow that much hair. Some boys may find that their hair doesn't grow very fast. Or they may find that the hair on the top may grow quickly, while the middle grows slower. This can be very frustrating if all your son's friends are wearing cornrows or twists and his hair is still too short to do either style. In the meantime, Hill suggests having your son's barber shape up the longer part of his hair to the length of his shorter hair.

10 Hair Problems

WHEN DADDY BRAIDS

When Kamaria and Gabrielle were babies, they had a lot of hair and it was very straight. Then Kamaria's hair just changed when she was seven months old. It just went crazy. So my wife and I would do Afro puffs, because it was easy.

I could do Afro puffs but not well. I had two daughters and I wanted to learn how to do their hair because I was their father. I don't think mothers should always have to do the hair.

But when I tried, the girls' hair would never stay straight. It never looked neat and it was frizzy around the edges. All I had to do is show Kamaria a brush and she would start crying.

One day I read an article about a braiding class at Prince Georges' Community College and I signed up for the class. The class was full of beauticians who were trying to learn how to braid. So I was one of the slowest people in the class. But I don't regret it at all. I can't do a lot of fancy styles, but I can do some simple plaits and some braids.

Now that my wife and I are divorced, I make it a point when I have my daughters to set aside Saturday night as the girls' hair night. I wash their hair, condition it, and braid it. It's a way for me to bond with my girls. I think they share more with me now because we have these braiding sessions.

It's funny to see their faces when their hair is done. They get in the mirror and look at themselves. They know they look good. Hair is important in the Black community and it will always be that way. And as time goes on, I think you will see more and more brothers learning how to braid their girls' hair.

—TODD BEAMON

Remember that braiding job you got that gave you a headache so bad that you had to go home and take two aspirins? Or the time you looked at your daughter's "nappy head" and decided that eight weeks was way too long to wait for a touch-up? And nothing you do seems to work on that dandruff on your son's scalp? These are hair and scalp conditions that may have to be treated by a doctor.

Good grooming is important to having healthy hair. Eating a healthy diet also plays a part in having hair that looks good. But sometimes our children's hair can be severely affected by chemicals or by a fungal infection. Here are some hair and scalp conditions to look out for:

Hair Breakage

Dr. Valerie Callender sees a lot of girls whose hair has been damaged by relaxers. If relaxers are not used properly, the chemicals can damage the cuticle and cause the hair to break off. Relaxers that weren't applied properly can also cause scabs on the scalp. "Usually the moms have used the regular or superstrength relaxer when they should have used mild," Callender says. "Or they used the 'kiddie perm' and the perm didn't get the hair straight enough. So Mom puts the relaxer on a second time."

Treatment

Stop relaxing the hair. More touch-ups will cause only more damage to the hair. For severe damage, the girls may have to consider cutting the hair off and wearing their hair as a short Afro until the hair can grow back. Braids and twists can be worn for several weeks at a time, so hair can rest. These hairstyles also reduce the chances for more hair breakage because they don't require daily combing and brushing. Apply conditioner to the hair and a topical antibiotic ointment to the scalp.

Ringworm or Tinea Capitis

Ringworm is caused by a fungus and is highly contagious. It is often spread from combs, brushes, and hats. It can also come from animals, dogs, and cats. Ringworm is frequently mistaken for dandruff.

Treatment

See a dermatologist who will prescribe an antifungal that is taken orally. If it is not treated, ringworm can

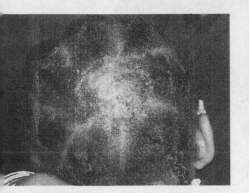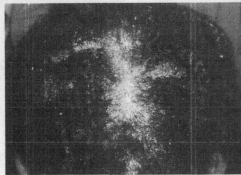

spread to other parts of the body or lead to alopecia or hair loss.

Alopecia

Alopecia is a medical term for hair loss. But traction alopecia can be prevented because it is caused by wearing or pulling the hair too tight. Usually it occurs at the forehead, where hair is braided or pulled too tightly.

Try to avoid braids that are braided too tightly. Your child shouldn't have a headache after her cornrows or extensions are put in her head.

Also avoid having your child wear ponytails all the time. Ponytails are a quick and easy hairdo. But don't put your child's hair in ponytails every day because this hairstyle could also lead to hair loss.

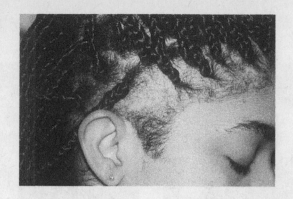

Wearing hair extensions that are too heavy can also cause hair breakage and loss.

Treatment

Avoid braiding or pulling the hair too tightly. Traction alopecia can be reversed, but if you continue to let your child wear the same hairstyle, the hair loss can be permanent. (Just think of all those ladies whose hairline start at their ears instead of their forehead!)

Alopecia Areata

Alopecia areata starts as small, coin-sized, smooth bald patches on the scalp. Some children have only a few patches on their scalp and the hair may grow back relatively quickly. A doctor can prescribe cortisone treatments for alopecia areata. In more severe cases of this, called alopecia totalis, a child's hair follicles are mistaken-

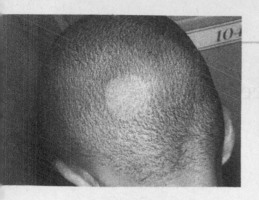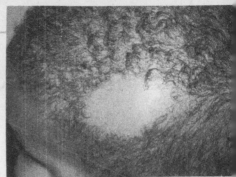

ly attacked by their white blood cells and it leads to total
hair loss.

Treatment

Please see your dermatologist for both conditions. The
National Alopecia Areata Foundation also has a good
homepage for more information, www.naaf.org.

Trichotillomania

This condition is caused by children who constantly
tug or pull on their hair. Often children pull out
clumps of their own hair.

Treatment

Trichotillomania is a psychological condition
requires counseling. Please see your doctor for
information.

Hair Resources

Blackkidshair.com. The companion website to this book offers more hair-care tips and styles.

Bailey, Diane Carol. *Natural Hair Care and Braiding*. New York: Milady Books, 1998.

Bonner, Britteneum Lonnice. *Plaited Glory: For Colored Girls Who've Considered Braids, Locks, and Twists*. New York: Three Rivers Press, 1996.

Ferrell, Pamela. *Kids Talk Hair: An Instruction Book for Grown-Ups*. Washington: Cornrows & Co. Publishing, 1999.

Herron, Carolivia. *I Love My Hair*. New York: Alfred A. Knopf, 1997.

hooks, bell. *Happy to Be Nappy*. New York: Hyperion Press, 1999.

Mastalia, Francesco and Alfonse Pagano. *Dreads*. New York: Artisan, 1999.

Yarbrough, Camille. *Nappy Hair*. New York: Putnam & Grossett Group, 1979.